T0249443

Winter Trauma

Editor

MARGARET M. ECKLUND

CRITICAL CARE NURSING CLINICS OF NORTH AMERICA

www.ccnursing.theclinics.com

Consulting Editor
JAN FOSTER

December 2012 • Volume 24 • Number 4

ELSEVIER

Elsevier Inc., 1600 John F. Kennedy Blvd., Suite 1800, Philadelphia, PA 19103-2899

http://www.theclinics.com

CRITICAL CARE NURSING CLINICS OF NORTH AMERICA Volume 24, Number 4
December 2012 ISSN 0899-5885, ISBN-13: 978-1-4557-4906-5

Editor: Katie Saunders
Developmental Editor: Donald Mumford

Critical Care Nursing Clinics of North America (ISSN 0899-5885) is published quarterly by Elsevier Inc., 360 Park Avenue South, New York, NY 10010-1710. Months of issue are March, June, September, and December. Business and Editorial Offices: 1600 John F. Kennedy Blvd., Suite 1800, Philadelphia, PA 19103-2899. Periodicals postage paid at New York, NY and additional mailing offices. Subscription prices are $144.00 per year for US individuals, $296.00 per year for US institutions, $76.00 per year for US students and residents, $192.00 per year for Canadian individuals, $371.00 per year for Canadian institutions, $219.00 per year for international individuals, $371.00 per year for international institutions and $111.00 per year for Canadian and foreign students/residents. To receive student/resident rate, orders must be accompanied by name of affiliated institution, data of term, and the *signature* of program/residency coordinator on institution letterhead. Orders will be billed at individual rate until proof of status is received. Foreign air speed delivery is included in all *Clinics* subscription prices. All prices are subject to change without notice. **POSTMASTER:** Send address changes to *Critical Care Nursing Clinics of North America*, Elsevier Health Sciences Division, Subscription Customer Service, 3251 Riverport Lane, Maryland Heights, MO 63043. **Customer Service: 1-800-654-2452 (US and Canada); 314-447-8871 (outside US and Canada). Fax: 314-447-8029. E-mail: JournalsCustomerService-usa@elsevier.com (for print support) and JournalsOnlineSupport-usa@elsevier.com (for online support).**

Reprints. For copies of 100 or more of articles in this publication, please contact the Commercial Reprints Department, Elsevier Inc., 360 Park Avenue South, New York, New York, 10010-1710; Tel.: (212) 633-3813, Fax: (212) 462-1935, and E-mail: reprints@elsevier.com.

Critical Care Nursing Clinics of North America is covered in *MEDLINE/PubMed (Index Medicus), International Nursing Index, Nursing Citation Index, Cumulative Index to Nursing and Allied Health Literature, and RNdex Top 100.*

Printed and bound by CPI Group (UK) Ltd, Croydon, CR0 4YY

Transferred to digital print 2012

Contributors

CONSULTING EDITOR

JAN FOSTER, PhD, RN, CNS
Texas Woman's University, College of Nursing, Houston, Texas

GUEST EDITOR

MARGARET M. ECKLUND, MS, RN, CCRN, ACNP-BC
Nurse Practitioner, Pulmonary Medicine–Progressive Care, Rochester General Health System, Hill Haven Nursing and Rehabilitation, Rochester, New York

AUTHORS

CHRISTIE E. ARTUSO, EdD, RN, CNRN
Director, Neuroscience Services, Providence Alaska Medical Center, Anchorage, Alaska

LYNN C. AYERS, MS, APRN, CCRN
Clinical Nurse Specialist, Rochester General Hospital, Rochester, New York

ZARA R. BRENNER, MS, RN-BC, ACNS-BC
Care Manager, Care Management, Surgical Intensive Care Unit, Rochester General Hospital, Rochester, New York; Assistant Professor, The College at Brockport, State University of New York, Brockport, New York

MARCELLA L. CARR, LPN
Registered Nurse Student, Finger Lakes Health College of Nursing, Geneva, New York

LORI A. DAMBAUGH, BSN, RN, DNP-C
Clinical Nurse Specialist, Progressive Pulmonary Care Unit, Department of Nursing, Rochester General Hospital; St. John Fisher College, Wegmans School of Nursing, Rochester, New York

MARGARET M. ECKLUND, MS, RN, CCRN, ACNP-BC
Nurse Practitioner, Pulmonary Care, Rochester General Health System, Rochester, New York

CHRISTINE R. ERNST, DNP, RN, FNP-BC
Oregon Health & Science University, Portland, Oregon

TERI LYNN KISS, RN, MS, MSSW, CCRN
Director, Medical Unit 2 South, Fairbanks Memorial Hospital, Fairbanks, Alaska

MAUREEN E. KRENZER, MS, RN, ACNS-BC
Clinical Nurse Specialist, Department of Nursing, Rochester General Hospital, Rochester, New York

ARLEEN B. MILLER, MS, APRN, CCRN
Clinical Nurse Specialist, Rochester General Hospital, Rochester, New York

ASHLIE ROBERTS, MS, APRN, CCRN
Clinical Nurse Specialist, Newark Wayne Community Hospital, Newark, New York

MICHAEL S. SMITH
Pulmonary Care, Rochester General Health System, Rochester, New York

DEBORAH C. STAMPS, EdD, RN, GNP, NE, BC
Vice President, Chief Nursing Officer, Newark Wayne Community Hospital, Newark, New York

EMILY ELIZABETH VERGER, RN, BSN
Clinical Nurse II, Neurology and General Pediatrics, Children's Hospital of Philadelphia, Philadelphia, Pennsylvania

JUDY TRIVITS VERGER, RN, PhD, CRNP
Director, Pediatric Critical Care and Neonatal Nurse Practitioner Programs; Director, Neonatal and Pediatric Clinical Nurse Specialist Programs, School of Nursing, University of Pennsylvania; APN Manager, Critical Care – Sedation/Radiology, Children's Hospital of Philadelphia, Philadelphia, Pennsylvania

GARY WAHL, MD
Department of Pulmonary Medicine, Rochester General Health System, Rochester General Hospital, Rochester, New York

ALEXANDRA V. YAMSHCHIKOV, MD
Assistant Professor, Infectious Diseases Unit, Rochester General Hospital, University of Rochester School of Medicine, Rochester, New York

Contents

requires symptomatic treatment alone. Complicated cases develop severe dehydration and hypovolemia, requiring the skills of critical care nurses to meet the challenges of care. This article addresses diagnosis and prevention strategies.

Judy Trivits Verger and Emily Elizabeth Verger

Respiratory syncytial virus is a highly infectious virus that commonly causes bronchiolitis and leads to high morbidity and a low, but important, incidence of mortality. Supportive therapy is the foundation of management. Hydration/nutrition and respiratory support are important evidence-based interventions. For children with severe disease, continuous positive airway pressure or mechanical ventilation may be necessary. Ribavirin may be used for treatment of patients with severe disease. Palivizumab provides important ongoing immunoprophylaxis during epidemic months for high-risk infants. Caregiver education and incorporating an explanation of all therapies and anticipatory guidance, including strategies for reducing the risk of infection, are vital.

Lori A. Dambaugh

The influenza virus is a significant cause of morbidity and mortality each year in the United States, and is a major public health problem. Individuals aged 65 years and older comprise a sizeable population subgroup at high risk of infection and subsequent complications. Although influenza may cause substantial morbidity and mortality across the age spectrum, it becomes particularly problematic for those older than 65. This article presents an overview of influenza, with a focus on how the influenza virus has particular implications for the geriatric population.

Teri Lynn Kiss

Frostbite, a preventable cold-weather injury, occurs when the skin temperature cools to below 0°C with the formation of extracellular ice crystals. On rewarming, an inflammatory response develops, contributing to ischemia and tissue loss. The severity of injury depends on the temperature, duration of exposure, and amount and depth of frozen tissue. Environmental, individual, behavioral, and physiologic factors increase susceptibility to cold. Rapid rewarming and watchful waiting remains the mainstay of treatment. Prevention can be accomplished through increasing public awareness of the adverse effects of cold exposure, and recognizing and mitigating the risks associated with the development of frostbite.

Christie E. Artuso

Rural trauma during winter months in Alaska requires a coordinated highly skilled approach for rescue, recovery, resuscitation, and transport to distant tertiary care centers. Clinicians in this state face travel delays, extreme weather conditions, and unique transport scenarios. Early assessment and resuscitation may focus more on minimizing delays than on the traditional ABCs of emergency medicine. Clinical evaluation and treatment is also impacted by subzero temperatures, hypothermia, and prolonged exposure. Mechanical and equipment malfunctions can complicate decisions and further add to the challenges faced by medical teams who respond and deliver care in the vast wilderness of this state.

This article discusses a woman who collapsed and landed in a puddle of water in a park near a horse trail. Her rescue and resuscitation started an extraordinary effort by her body to heal from multiple insults. This case study highlights the diagnosis and support of polymicrobial pneumonia secondary to near drowning and the multisystem complications throughout the 3-month hospitalization. It highlights the evidence for treatment of the polymicrobial nature of submersion injury, acute lung injury, and benefits of progressive mobility. Social media as a tool for the family's communication and coping are also discussed.

CRITICAL CARE NURSING CLINICS OF NORTH AMERICA

**DOWNLOAD
Free App!**

Review Articles
THE CLINICS

NOW AVAILABLE FOR YOUR iPhone and iPad

Preface

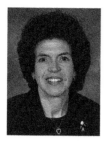

Margaret M. Ecklund, MS, RN, CCRN, ACNP-BC
Guest Editor

The color of springtime is in the flowers; the color of winter is in the imagination.
— *Terri Guillemets.*

The term "winter" provokes different images depending on where you live. Acute and critical care nurses face a variety of difficulties in their patients, who span a wide range of acuity. Thus, this issue's topic of Winter Trauma provided a unique challenge to coordinate. The concept was broad enough to be creative with the season, climate, and health issues relative to winter. Authors were able to retell their stories and analyze how individuals respond to winter health issues. I am pleased to present a range of authors from across the country. The majority of authors are colleagues from the Rochester, New York area. Within the group of writers, many have diverse writing experience and mentored fellow novice writers. There are also several second-generation nurses: daughters who are now nurse authors.

The *Critical Care Nursing Clinics of North America* begin by exploring seasonal issues in the winter months. Ernst explores depression relative to the season, with a case study presentation to stimulate clinician awareness of depression as a comorbidity to critical illness. The Holiday Heart Syndrome, with the incidence of cardiac arrhythmias and associated symptoms, is a documented phenomenon nationwide. Stamps and Carr describe the evidence relative to this syndrome.

Climate challenges in northern regions include diminished amounts of sunshine. This may suggest a deficiency of Vitamin D. Brenner, Ayers, Miller, and Roberts present a comprehensive discussion of Vitamin D and the role of deficiency in the care of the critically ill patient. The recommendations are a subject of debate among health care professionals.

Seasonal effects of communicable diseases may be relative to being confined to the indoors. Viral gastroenteritis is described by Krenzer with evidence and implications. For children, RSV can be a peril for critical illness. The Vergers describe the challenges of RSV. Influenza is associated with winter months across the country. Dambaugh provides a comprehensive overview of influenza and the implications of vaccinations.

Crit Care Nurs Clin N Am 24 (2012) ix–x
http://dx.doi.org/10.1016/j.ccell.2012.07.010
0899-5885/12/$ – see front matter © 2012 Elsevier Inc. All rights reserved.

ccnursing.theclinics.com

Conditions can arise from severe forms of weather. Frostbite, rural trauma, and near drowning are winter challenges. Frostbite, a cold weather challenge, is described by Kiss, an Alaskan nurse. She explores the diagnosis and treatment options for various stages of frostbite. Artruso, also an Alaskan nurse, explores the challenges of managing trauma in the rural setting. She elaborates on the nature of various accidents and the trauma system to meet the needs in remote settings.

On a personal note, the final topic of near drowning goes beyond the clinical expertise of a case of near drowning to the human response to critical illness and family response. This is a collaborative case study, with the physiological implications described by my physician colleagues Wahl and Yamshchikov, and with the personal reflections by Smith, on behalf of the patient and family. We demonstrated how social media are used as a reflection and processing tool for family.

I am grateful to have had this opportunity provided to me from Jan Foster! This issue is edited in memorial tribute to my writing and professional mentors: Karen Carlson, who encouraged my professional writing; Sharon Connor, who nurtured my AACN leadership. I wish to recognize Zara Brenner, who has always supported and encouraged my professional contributions.

I present to you the work of authors who shared their time and talent to provide acute and critical readers a great discussion of winter health challenges.

Margaret M. Ecklund, MS, RN, CCRN, ACNP-BC
Pulmonary Medicine–Progressive Care
Rochester General Health System
Hill Haven Nursing and Rehabilitation
1425 Portland Avenue
Rochester, NY 14621, USA

E-mail address:
Margaret.ecklund@rochestergeneral.org

Winter Depression and Diabetes

Christine R. Ernst, DNP, RN, FNP-BC

KEYWORDS

- Depression • Type 2 diabetes mellitus • Seasonal affective disorder • Seasonality

KEY POINTS

- Depression is a common disorder that is often associated with the winter season.
- There is a link between type 2 diabetes mellitus and depression.
- Seasonal affective disorder (SAD) is a specifier of major depressive disorder and bipolar disorders, with recurring seasonal patterns of onset and remission. Depressive symptoms occur most often in the winter.
- The SAD criteria are complex, and there exists a level of skepticism about the disorder from the medical community.

PURPOSE

Depression is a common mood disorder faced by many people in the United States and worldwide, with often damaging effects. According to a publication from the Centers for Disease Control and Prevention, more than 5% of (or more than 1 in 20) Americans older than 12 years suffer from current depression.[1] In addition, the World Health Organization[2] recognized depression as the leading cause of disability internationally among people from birth to age 59 years. Although depression can occur at any time of the year, it is commonly associated with the winter season, with terms such as the "winter blues" or "winter depression."

Seasonal affective disorder (SAD), a subtype or specifier of major depressive disorder and bipolar I or II disorders, has recurring seasonal patterns of onset and remission, with depressive symptoms most often occurring in the winter, called fall-onset.[3] Similarly, studies have shown that people with nonseasonal depression may exhibit worsening symptoms in the winter months. Furthermore, many people develop depressive symptoms in the winter that do not meet the severity of SAD criteria, but still experience significant difficulty performing their daily activities, a condition termed subsyndromal SAD (S-SAD).[4,5]

Depression can often occur concurrently with chronic illnesses, such as type 2 diabetes mellitus.[6] Diabetics with comorbid depression are at increased risk for complications, poorer quality of life, and increased mortality.[7–9] Despite the cause

The author has nothing to disclose.
Oregon Health & Science University, 3181 SW Sam Jackson Park Road, Portland, OR 97239, USA
E-mail address: ernstc@ohsu.edu

Crit Care Nurs Clin N Am 24 (2012) 509–518
http://dx.doi.org/10.1016/j.ccell.2012.07.006
0899-5885/12/$ – see front matter © 2012 Elsevier Inc. All rights reserved.

of depression, it is of great importance for clinicians, such as advanced practice nurses, to treat or prevent the mood disorder in these patients. The purpose of this case report is to examine the literature for evidence-based diagnosis and management guidelines for those with type 2 diabetes who experience winter onset or worsening of depression.

BACKGROUND

Major depressive disorder affects approximately 6.7% of adults in the United States, with a lifetime prevalence of 16.5%[10,11]; however, people with diabetes have twice the risk for depression than the general population, and lifetime prevalence of 28% for major depression.[6] Prevalence rates for SAD are varied in the literature. Studies have shown rates as low as 1% and as high as 12%, depending on the sample population and method of diagnosis. S-SAD, a milder form of SAD, has also been reported with prevalence rates from 10% to 20%. No studies have reported the prevalence of SAD or seasonality of depressed mood in the type 1 or type 2 diabetic population.[10,11]

As in major depressive disorder, the incidence for SAD is greater among females than males.[10] Depression is also more prevalent in the female population of diabetics.[6] There are limited data regarding the prevalence of SAD among age and racial groups,[12] although onset favors the third decade.[3]

Although the etiology of SAD is not fully understood, some researchers have demonstrated a link between photoperiod (light/dark cycle) and SAD because the prevalence of SAD seems to increase in regions with less daylight in the winter, otherwise known as the latitude hypothesis. Some have found evidence to the contrary; however, the effectiveness of bright-light therapy in fall-onset SAD lends credence to the latitude theory.[13] Despite the common belief that bad weather correlates with saddening mood, researchers have delineated that meteorologic conditions, such as temperature, duration of sunshine, and duration of rainfall are not associated with mood variation. Nevertheless, depressive symptoms, whether they are attributable to SAD or nonseasonal depression, are more prevalent in the winter months.[4,13]

SIGNIFICANCE

The prevalence of diabetes has grown substantially over the last 40 years in the United States.[14] Approximately 25 million Americans currently have some form of diabetes.[15] Type 2 diabetes represents 90% to 95% of all diagnosed cases. As providers, this growth not only implies increased treatment for glycemic control but other comorbid conditions as well.

Anderson and colleagues[6] reported that odds of depression in both type 1 and type 2 diabetics was twice that in nondiabetics (odds ratio = 2.0, 95% confidence interval 1.8–2.2). Confirmatory data was later published on type 2 diabetics.[16] In addition, research has indicated that individuals with type 2 diabetes and depression are at greater risk for poor glycemic control and increased complications, have increased costs of care, poorer quality of life, and increased mortality compared with their nondepressed counterparts.[7–9]

SAD and S-SAD can be detrimental to a diabetic. The symptoms often present in these disorders are similar to those in atypical depression, another subtype of major depressive disorder. Symptoms include fatigue, hypersomnia, increased appetite with a propensity toward carbohydrate craving, and weight gain.[5] These symptoms can easily exacerbate glycemic control in a patient with type 2 diabetes, whose core regimen revolves around carbohydrate control and adequate physical activity.

With the epidemic growth of type 2 diabetes in the general population, providers such as advanced practice nurses should expect to be faced with increasing health challenges in these patients, such as screening and treating comorbid depression. Although rates for SAD among diabetics are not currently available, it is likely that depressive disorders in diabetics have seasonal components similar to those of the general population. Because of the detrimental impacts of depression among patients with type 2 diabetes, awareness of evidence-based diagnosis and treatment options for SAD or seasonal worsening of depression is necessary.

KEY CONCEPTS

Although notions of seasonality date back to Hippocrates, Rosenthal and colleagues[17] were the first to delineate SAD in the modern literature. Since that time, researchers have struggled to define diagnostic criteria as well as prove its validity as a distinct disorder.[18] Skeptics from the medical community have asserted that SAD is merely an exaggerated form of a seasonal mood variation that occurs in the general population.[5] Others doubt its distinction as a separate entity because it presents with features similar to atypical depression or, further, that the "distinction from other types of recurrent depression is irrelevant."[19] However, evidence showing the unique effectiveness of bright-light therapy in SAD patients supports the continued use of the concept, if only to justify management options.[19]

Under the *Diagnostic and Statistical Manual of Mental Disorders* (Fourth Edition, Text Revised) (DSM-IV-TR) criteria, SAD is currently considered a subtype or "specifier" of major depressive disorder, as with other subtypes: melancholic, atypical, catatonic, and postpartum.[3] The seasonal pattern specifier can also be applied to bipolar I or bipolar II disorder.[3] For the purposes of this case report, only major depressive disorder is discussed.

A diagnosis for major depressive disorder is based on the criteria listed in **Box 1**. SAD specifier criteria can be found in **Box 2**. The key differentiating factor between recurrent nonseasonal depression and SAD is failed remission from depressive symptoms in the summer for nonseasonal depression.

EVIDENCE RELEVANT TO THE CASE

Seasonality has been studied in the diabetic population. Several researchers have elucidated a seasonal variation in hemoglobin A_{1c} (HbA_{1c}) values, revealing a worsening of glycemic control in the winter.[20] Studies on blood glucose levels and insulin sensitivity have also shown similar findings.[20–23] Although causality remains unclear, the literature supports a relationship between worsening glycemic control and increased depressive symptoms.[24,25]

What causes seasonal variation in glycemic control is uncertain. Some have argued that these seasonal physiologic changes seen in humans are leftover adaptive characteristics for survival, expressed in other mammals too, such as hibernation.[26] Though at one time beneficial, these physiologic changes are detrimental over time to the modern human, and may be contributing to the presence of chronic diseases including type 2 diabetes. Of note, the incidence of diabetes increases in the winter season,[27] perhaps because of the spike of metabolic changes in the winter months.

Others assert that seasonal variation in glycemic control may be related to environmental conditions, such as diet and exercise, which may fluctuate over the seasons. Obesity is a key predictor of insulin resistance,[28] and therefore glycemic control. Several studies from the United States have indicated a seasonal variation in body weight, with increases over the winter holidays,[28] which may increase risk for depression.

Box 1
DSM-IV-TR criteria for a major depressive episode

A. Five or more of the following symptoms have been present during the same 2-week period, nearly every day, and represent a change from previous functioning.

At least *one* of the following:

- Depressed mood
- Markedly diminished interest or pleasure in all, or almost all, activities

Other symptoms:

- Significant weight loss while not dieting, weight gain, or decrease/increase in appetite
- Insomnia or hypersomnia
- Psychomotor agitation or retardation
- Fatigue or loss of energy
- Feelings of worthlessness or excessive or inappropriate guilt
- Diminished ability to think or concentrate, or indecisiveness
- Recurrent thoughts of death, recurrent suicidal ideation without a specific plan, or a suicide attempt or a specific plan of committing suicide

B. The symptoms do not meet criteria for a Mixed Episode

C. The symptoms cause clinically significant distress or impairment in social, occupational, or other important areas of functioning

D. The symptoms are not due to the direct physiologic effects of substance or a general medical condition

E. The symptoms are not better accounted for by bereavement (except after the loss of a loved one), the symptoms persist for longer than 2 months or are characterized by marked functional impairment, morbid preoccupation with worthlessness, suicidal ideation, psychotic symptoms, or psychomotor retardation

Adapted from American Psychological Association. Diagnostic and statistical manual of mental disorders. 4th edition, Text Revision. Washington, DC: APA; 2000; with permission.

Box 2
DSM-IV-TR criteria for seasonal pattern specifier

A. Regular temporal relationship between the onset of major depressive episodes in Bipolar I or Bipolar II Disorder or Major Depressive Disorder, recurrent, and a particular time of the year unrelated to obvious season-related psychosocial stressors

B. Full remissions (or a change from depression to mania or hypomania) also occur at a characteristic time of the year

C. Two major depressive episodes meeting criteria A and B in the last 2 years and no nonseasonal episodes in the same period

D. Seasonal major depressive episodes substantially outnumber the nonseasonal episodes over the individual's lifetime

Adapted from American Psychological Association. Diagnostic and statistical manual of mental disorders. 4th edition, Text Revision. Washington, DC: APA; 2000; with permission.

One study reported that weather had modest effects on physical activity, decreasing participants' total daily steps by up to 20%.[29] Several other studies have shown a reduction in daily steps in the fall and winter in patients with type 2 diabetes.[30,31] Lysy and colleagues[32] reported a relationship between physical inactivity and depression in adults with type 2 diabetes, stating that physically inactive people are more likely to be depressed and vice versa, thereby increasing diabetics' risk for depression in the winter.

There is a dearth of literature regarding SAD in diabetic patients. A case study reported an increase in insulin sensitivity after bright-light therapy in diabetic patients with SAD. This finding is likely due to the suppressing effect that light therapy has on the secretion of melatonin, a hormone that otherwise diminishes insulin sensitivity.[33] More research is needed on diabetic patients with SAD to confirm the possible role of light therapy in this population.

Screening and diagnosis for SAD remains somewhat ambiguous. The Seasonal Pattern Assessment Questionnaire (SPAQ),[34] an instrument used to identify patients with SAD, has been used widely in the literature for epidemiologic studies, but has performed poorly on statistical tests of sensitivity, specificity, positive predictive value, and test-retest reliability.[35] It focuses on periodicity of atypical symptoms but does not screen for major depression criteria, whereas the DSM-IV-TR and the International Classification of Diseases criteria focus more on seasonal recurrence of major depression, regardless of presentation. In addition, there are varying guidelines as to how many repeated episodes of seasonal depression must occur and how many nonseasonal episodes are permitted to fit seasonal specifier diagnostic criteria, all of which can be perplexing to the clinician.[35]

Light therapy is generally accepted as the first-line treatment for SAD,[36,37] although the National Institute for Health and Clinical Excellence[38] guidelines did not find sufficient evidence to support its use. Light therapy was recently shown to be effective in nonseasonal depression as well.[39] Of note, exercise was as effective as light therapy and was more effective than light therapy in seasonal and nonseasonal depression patients, respectively.[39]

Selective serotonin reuptake inhibitors (SSRIs) are recognized as the first-line agent for pharmacotherapy in seasonal and nonseasonal depression.[5,40] Fluoxetine, an SSRI, has proved to be effective in treating both seasonal and nonseasonal depression.[40] In addition, fluoxetine was efficacious in reducing depression in the diabetic population, although combined pharmacotherapy and psychotherapy with self-care education for diabetic patients were most successful at also increasing glycemic control.[41]

A clinical response is generally defined as a greater than or equal to 50% reduction in depressive symptoms, which should be reached within 2 to 4 weeks after initiating therapy.[40] Patients should be continued on their medication at the acute-treatment dose for at least 6 months after remission.[36] Preventive therapy, such as continuous pharmacotherapy or strategies to maintain activity levels in the winter, should be considered.

CONTEXT FOR CASE

The following case report describes a woman with type 2 diabetes who presented to her primary care provider in early February with complaints of depressed mood. She exhibited some classic risk factors and symptoms of SAD described in the literature, but given the lack of research regarding SAD in diabetics, the clinician had to use careful consideration to drive the plan of care. The woman was screened for current depression and treated according to evidence-based guidelines.

CASE PRESENTATION

Ruth, a 65-year-old Caucasian woman, presented to her family nurse practitioner for her 3-month diabetic checkup. During the course of the visit, the patient stated that she had been "feeling down" for the past month. She had spent most of the last couple months at home watching television. She had not been motivated to see anyone or do anything. She stated, "I always get like this in the winter."

She further described that she was tired all the time, sleeping for up to 14 hours a day. She overate most days of the week. She had trouble concentrating on things, such as watching the news on TV. She admitted that she had not been checking her blood sugars regularly and occasionally forgot to take her medication. She denied any current or past anxiety, mania, or thoughts of self harm. All other review of systems was negative.

Ruth had suffered from depression in the past, for which she had been on medication, but was not currently taking any antidepressants. She had type 2 diabetes of 22 years' duration, and developed diabetic retinopathy and diabetic neuropathy. She also had hypertension, hyperlipidemia, osteoarthritis, and was obese.

Her family history included a mother and sister with depression. Her mother also had type 2 diabetes and died of a stroke at age 72 years. Her father had hypertension and coronary artery disease. He died of a myocardial infarction at age 68 years. She had 2 grown children who were alive and well.

Ruth was a retired city worker. She was a widow and had lived alone for about 5 years since her husband's passing, after 42 years of marriage. Her children lived out of state. She was originally from California, but moved to the Pacific Northwest with her husband after high school. She had a 20-pack year history of tobacco use, but had quit. She did not drink any alcohol or use other street drugs. Her diet was not well balanced, and tended to be carbohydrate heavy. Her activity level was restricted by her obesity, osteoarthritis, and peripheral neuropathy, but she could go for half-mile walks if the weather was nice. She was afraid of walking alone in the dark in her neighborhood and did not like to be in the wet and cold weather. Financially she had limited resources.

Ruth's medication included: metformin, 1000 mg by mouth twice a day; glargine, 35 units subcutaneously at bedtime; hydrochlorothiazide, 25 mg daily; lisinopril, 20 mg daily; atorvastatin, 40 mg daily; and pregabalin, 75 mg twice a day. She also took hydrocodone/acetaminophen 5/500, 2 tablets, 3 times daily as needed for her joint pain.

Ruth lacked a strong support system, with her husband deceased and her children out of state. Although she attended regular religious services every Sunday, she generally did not partake in any other activities outside her house other than running errands. Her mobility could be limited on some days because of her osteoarthritis and peripheral neuropathy, which also prohibited her from wanting to leave her home; however, she was able to perform her activities of daily living without assistance.

On physical examination Ruth was an obese, tired-appearing woman who looked older than her stated age. Her vitals on her day of visit were: blood pressure 140/80 mm Hg; pulse 86 beats per minute; respirations 20 breaths per minute. She was 5 ft 5 inches (1.65 m) tall; weight was 199 pounds (90.2 kg) with a body mass index of 33.1 kg/m^2. She had gained 12 pounds (5.4 kg) since her last visit in October, about 3 months ago. Cardiovascular and respiratory examinations were normal. Thyroid was normal on palpation. Diabetic foot examination revealed decreased sensation to light touch, but vibratory sense was intact bilaterally. The patient scored a 17 on the Patient Health Questionnaire (PHQ-9) screening for depression, and cited her symptoms as "very difficult" to manage, which indicated Major Depressive Disorder.

A SPAQ was not available at the time of examination; however, the clinician asked the patient to recall previous episodes of depression. Her first episode of depression was when she was 23 years old. Most episodes happened in the winter, but not every year. She did not remember having a major depressive episode last year. She also generally reported having better moods in the summer, when she could get outside, but had depression last all year on previous occasions. She indicated that her appetite, especially for carbohydrates, and sleep usually increase substantially in the winter months, as well as her weight.

Laboratory results from this visit included an HbA_{1c} of 9.9%, up from 7.2% in the fall. The American Diabetes Association (2012)[42] recommends that HbA_{1c} be less than 7.0% for most nonpregnant adults. A complete set of laboratory tests were drawn 3 months previously, which revealed normal complete metabolic panel, except an elevated fasting glucose at 139 mg/dL (normal 70–100 mg/dL), a normal complete blood count, and lipids that were controlled. Thyroid-stimulating hormone was normal at 1.7 mIU/L (normal 0.5–5 mIU/L).

With this information, the nurse practitioner needed to make some critical decisions. Ruth was clearly struggling with her depression, as evidenced by her complaints coming into the office and her PHQ-9 score. She had also gained 12 pounds in 3 months and her HbA_{1c} had dramatically worsened. The patient had recalled repeated depressive episodes occurring during the winter season over her lifetime, but not in 2 consecutive years. She also experienced some depressive episodes in the summer, although her seasonal depressive episodes seemed to outnumber her nonseasonal ones. Nevertheless, according to the DSM-IV-TR criteria, she did not meet the seasonal specifier requirements.

The nurse practitioner considered use of bright-light therapy, based on the patient's depression history correlating with the winter season in a place of higher latitude and presence of atypical symptoms. However, the patient had diabetic retinopathy, which is a relative contraindication to bright-light therapy given the theoretical risk for bright light–induced eye toxicity.[5] The cost of obtaining a light box and concern for compliance with the therapy were also determining factors.

The nurse practitioner discussed possible treatment options with Ruth, including risks and benefits. The plan arrived at was a trial of antidepressants. Ruth recalled taking fluoxetine in the past with success, so this drug was selected for use. The patient was started on fluoxetine 20 mg daily, with plans for follow-up in 2 weeks. No adjustments to her diabetic medications were made because the patient was reportedly not taking her medication consistently. The patient was encouraged to resume her prior regimen and check her blood sugar daily before breakfast. Activity options were discussed, including walking at the local mall if the weather was poor or meeting with people from her faith community for social interaction. Other suggestions included counseling, behavior therapy, or mental health follow-up for investigative therapies aimed at SAD.

A 2-week follow-up visit revealed a happier Ruth. She was tolerating her fluoxetine well, and felt that she was doing better. Her PHQ-9 score at follow-up was 8. She was taking her medication as directed again, and fasting blood sugars were back down to below 140. She felt more motivated to be active during the day and was planning to join some social groups at her church. Another follow-up visit was scheduled for 10 weeks later to recheck her HbA_{1c} and reevaluate her depressive symptoms.

Summary of Case

This case depicts a patient with type 2 diabetes and a history of depression in the winter, a family history of depression, and current symptoms characteristic of atypical depression as well as worsening glycemic control. The nurse practitioner and patient decided to forgo the light therapy and restart antidepressants. The patient was also encouraged to resume diabetic self care to regain glycemic control and attempt to engage in other activities outside the house, to help improve moods. The patient was able to achieve interim success with the fluoxetine and felt motivated to take control of her diabetes as well as interact with others in her faith group.

SUMMARY

Winter depression, whether it is truly SAD, S-SAD, or worsening of recurrent or chronic depression, can be a challenge to diagnose and treat. In patients with type 2 diabetes, winter depression can prove especially difficult because of the potentially detrimental impact on glycemic control, as well as other serious sequelae. Although bright-light therapy is the hallmark treatment for SAD, extra caution must be exercised for diabetic patients given their risk for retinopathy. Overall, this patient responded well to an SSRI, and was able to regain some motivation to resume her diabetes regimen as well as her desire for social integration.

LESSONS LEARNED

Depression can have a potentially crippling effect on patients, including diabetics. As providers, it is common to hear patients complain that their depression worsens in the winter or that the cold weather negatively affects their moods. This case explored the seasonality of depression. The SAD criteria are complex and there exists a level of skepticism from the medical community regarding the disorder. Antidepressants and other therapies, however, can have a positive effect and reverse some of the adverse outcomes.

Within the acute care setting, SAD or worsening of depression in the winter among diabetics can be seen as comorbidities with more urgent critical needs. Patients may present to the emergency department with fatally high blood sugars or other complications attributable to uncontrolled diabetes. Detection and prevention of depression in patients with diabetes can be life altering. Depression screening tools should be considered in the acute care setting as a modality for identifying patients at risk.

REFERENCES

1. Pratt LA, Brody DJ. Depression in the United States household population, 2005-2006. NCHS Data Brief 2008;(7):1–8. Available at: http://www.cdc.gov/nchs/data/databriefs/db07.pdf. Accessed February 2, 2012.
2. World Health Organization. Global burden of disease: 2004 update. Geneva (Switzerland): WHO Press; 2008.
3. American Psychological Association. Diagnostic and statistical manual of mental disorders. 4th edition. Text Revision. Washington, DC: Author; 2000.
4. Oyane NM, Bjelland I, Pallesen S, et al. Seasonality is associated with anxiety and depression: the Hordaland health study. J Affect Disord 2008;105:147–55.
5. Westrin A, Lam RW. Seasonal affective disorder: a clinical update. Ann Clin Psychiatry 2007;19:239–46.
6. Anderson RJ, Freedland KE, Clouse RE, et al. The prevalence of comorbid depression in adults with diabetes: a meta-analysis. Diabetes Care 2001;24:1069–78.
7. Lin EH, Rutter CM, Katon W, et al. Depression and advanced complications of diabetes: a prospective cohort study. Diabetes Care 2010;33:264–9.

8. Verma SK, Luo N, Subramaniam M, et al. Impact of depression on health related quality of life in patients with diabetes. Ann Acad Med Singap 2010;39:913-7.
9. Williams LH, Rutter CM, Katon WJ, et al. Depression and incident diabetic foot ulcers: a prospective cohort study. Am J Med 2010;123:748-754.e3.
10. Kessler RC, Berglund P, Demler O, et al. Lifetime prevalence and age-of-onset distributions of DSM-IV disorders in the National Comorbidity Survey Replication. Arch Gen Psychiatry 2005;62:593-602.
11. Kessler RC, Chiu WT, Demler O, et al. Prevalence, severity, and comorbidity of 12-Month DSM-IV disorders in the National Comorbidity Survey Replication. Arch Gen Psychiatry 2005;62:617-27.
12. Partonen T, Lonnqvist J. Seasonal affective disorder. Lancet 1998;352:1369-74.
13. Huibers MJ, de Graaf LE, Peeters FP, et al. Does the weather make us sad? Meteorological determinants of mood and depression in the general population. Psychiatry Res 2010;180:143-6.
14. Centers for Disease Control and Prevention Division of Diabetes Translation. Long-term trends in diabetes. Atlanta (GA): U. S. Department of Health and Human Services, Centers for Disease Control and Prevention; 2010. Available at: http://www.cdc.gov/diabetes/statistics/slides/long_term_trends.pdf. Accessed February 2, 2012.
15. Centers for Disease Control and Prevention. National diabetes fact sheet: National estimates and general information on diabetes and prediabetes in the United States, 2011. Atlanta (GA): U. S. Department of Health and Human Services, Centers for Disease Control and Prevention; 2011. Available at: http://www.cdc.gov/diabetes/pubs/pdf/ndfs_2011.pdf. Accessed February 2, 2012.
16. Nouwen A, Winkley K, Twisk J, et al, European Depression in Diabetes (EDID) Research Consortium. Type 2 diabetes mellitus as a risk factor for the onset of depression: a systematic review and meta-analysis. Diabetologia 2010;53:2480-6.
17. Rosenthal NE, Sack DA, Gillin JC, et al. Seasonal affective disorder. A description of the syndrome and preliminary findings with light therapy. Arch Gen Psychiatry 1984;41:72-80.
18. Rosenthal NE. Issues for DSM-V: seasonal affective disorder and seasonality. Am J Psychiatry 2009;166:852-3.
19. Eagles JM. Light therapy and the management of winter depression. Adv Psychiatr Treat 2004;10:233-40.
20. Gikas A, Sotiropoulos A, Pastromas V, et al. Seasonal variation in fasting glucose and HbA1c in patients with type 2 diabetes. Prim Care Diabetes 2009;3:111-4.
21. Liang WW. Seasonal changes in preprandial glucose, A1C, and blood pressure in diabetic patients. Diabetes Care 2007;30:2501-2.
22. Kershenbaum A, Kershenbaum A, Tarabeia J, et al. Unraveling seasonality in population averages: an examination of seasonal variation in glucose levels in diabetes patients using a large population-based data set. Chronobiol Int 2011;28:352-60.
23. Isken F, Abraham U, Weickert MO, et al. Annual change in insulin sensitivity. Horm Metab Res 2011;43:720-2.
24. Richardson LK, Egede LE, Mueller M, et al. Longitudinal effects of depression on glycemic control in veterans with type 2 diabetes. Gen Hosp Psychiatry 2008;30:509-14.
25. Calhoun D, Beals J, Carter EA, et al. Relationship between glycemic control and depression among American Indians in the Strong Heart Study. J Diabetes Complications 2010;24:217-22.
26. Scott EM, Grant PJ. Neel revisited: the adipocyte, seasonality and type 2 diabetes. Diabetologia 2006;49:1462-6.

27. Doro P, Benko R, Matuz M, et al. Seasonality in the incidence of type 2 diabetes: a population-based study. Diabetes Care 2006;29:173.

28. Ma Y, Olendzki BC, Li W, et al. Seasonal variation in food intake, physical activity, and body weight in a predominantly overweight population. Eur J Clin Nutr 2006; 60:519–28.

29. Chan CB, Ryan DAJ, Tudor-Locke C. Relationship between objective measures of physical activity and weather: a longitudinal study. Int J Behav Nutr Phys Act 2006;3:21.

30. Dasgupta K, Chan C, Da Costa D, et al. Walking behaviour and glycemic control in type 2 diabetes: seasonal and gender differences—study design and methods. Cardiovasc Diabetol 2007;6:1.

31. Dasgupta K, Joseph L, Pilote L, et al. Daily steps are low year-round and dip lower in fall/winter: findings from a longitudinal diabetes cohort. Cardiovasc Diabetol 2010;9:81.

32. Lysy Z, Da Costa D, Dasgupta K. The association of physical activity and depression in type 2 diabetes. Diabet Med 2008;25:1133–41.

33. Nieuwenhuis RF, Spooren PF, Tilanus JJ. Less need for insulin, a surprising effect of phototherapy in insulin-dependent diabetes mellitus [abstract]. Tijdschr Psychiatr 2009;51:693–7 [in Dutch].

34. Thompson C, Stinson D, Fernandez M, et al. A comparison of normal, bipolar and seasonal affective disorder subjects using the Seasonal Pattern Assessment Questionnaire. J Affect Disord 1988;14:257–64.

35. Mersch PP, Vastenburg NC, Meesters Y, et al. The reliability and validity of the Seasonal Pattern Assessment Questionnaire: a comparison between patient groups. J Affect Disord 2004;80:209–19.

36. Anderson IM, Ferrier IN, Baldwin RC, et al. Evidence-based guidelines for treating depressive disorders with antidepressants: a revision of the 2000 British Association for Psychopharmacology guidelines. J Psychopharmacol 2008;22: 343–96.

37. Ravindran AV, Lam RW, Filteau MJ, et al, Canadian Network for Mood and Anxiety Treatments (CANMAT). Canadian Network for Mood and Anxiety Treatments (CANMAT) Clinical guidelines for the management of major depressive disorder in adults. V. Complementary and alternative medicine treatments. J Affect Disord 2009;117:S54–64.

38. National Institute for Health and Clinical Excellence. Depression: the treatment and management of depression in adults. Author; 2009. Available at: http://www.nice.org.uk/nicemedia/live/12329/45888/45888.pdf. Accessed February 2, 2012.

39. Lieverse R, Van Someren EJ, Nielen MM, et al. Bright light treatment in elderly patients with nonseasonal major depressive disorder: a randomized placebo-controlled trial. Arch Gen Psychiatry 2011;68:61–70.

40. Lam RW, Kennedy SH, Grigoriadis S, et al, Canadian Network for Mood and Anxiety Treatments (CANMAT). Canadian Network for Mood and Anxiety Treatments (CANMAT) clinical guidelines for the management of major depressive disorder in adults. III. Pharmacotherapy. J Affect Disord 2009;117:S26–43.

41. van der Feltz-Cornelis CM, Nuyen J, Stoop C, et al. Effect of interventions for major depressive disorder and significant depressive symptoms in patients with diabetes mellitus: a systematic review and meta-analysis. Gen Hosp Psychiatry 2010;32:380–95.

42. American Diabetes Association. Standards of medical care in diabetes—2012. Diabetes Care 2012;35:S11–63. http://dx.doi.org/10.2337/dc12-s011.

Holiday Season for a Healthy Heart

Deborah C. Stamps, EdD, RN, GNP, NE, BC[a],*, Marcella L. Carr, LPN[b]

KEYWORDS

- Holiday heart • Dysrhythmia • Atrial fibrillation • Alcohol consumption

KEY POINTS

- Holiday heart is defined as an acute cardiac arrhythmia or conduction disturbance associated with heavy intake of alcohol in persons with no known heart disease, and in whom the heart rhythm is restored to normal in the absence of alcohol.[1]
- Evidence has shown a higher cardiac mortality surrounding the Christmas and New Year holidays.
- There is an association between alcohol intake and atrial fibrillation.

INTRODUCTION

The holiday season, beginning around Thanksgiving and going through New Years' Day, can be a time of cheer, parties brimming with food and drink, and the pleasure of family and friend reunions. It can also be a stressful time and a time of too much eating, drinking, or money spent. These events along with other factors contribute to a spike in deaths due to heart disease during the holiday season.

Annually during the Christmas and New Year season, millions of Americans abruptly change their patterns of eating, drinking, exercising, working, and traveling. Large-scale behavioral changes may affect cardiac mortality. Some patients may inappropriately delay medical treatment until after the holidays. Family get-togethers, parties, and many hours indoors enjoying each other's company are all part of the holiday season. This time of year can often be a time of overeating and excessive alcohol consumption, both of which not only "pack on the pounds" but pose a risk for heart patients.

Many people tend to eat too much during the holiday season and unfortunately, holiday foods are usually high in fat, salt, or sugar. Patients with congestive heart

The authors have nothing to disclose.
[a] Nursing Administration, Newark Wayne Community Hospital, 1200 Driving Park Avenue, Newark, NY 14513, USA; [b] Student Nurse, Finger Lakes Health College of Nursing, 196 North Street, Geneva, NY 14456, USA
* Corresponding author.
E-mail address: Debbie.stamps@rochestergeneral.org

Crit Care Nurs Clin N Am 24 (2012) 519–525
http://dx.doi.org/10.1016/j.ccell.2012.07.007

failure (HF) who eat foods high in salt content can cause exacerbation of HF. People with diabetes who eat foods high in sugar content can increase blood sugar levels, and hypertensive individuals who eat foods high in salt content can increase their blood pressure. The risk of "holiday heart" for an otherwise healthy adult is higher at this time. According to Sterner and Keough,[2] holiday heart syndrome is a condition in which people that do not have heart disease suddenly develop a temporary dysrhythmia. The irregular heartbeat usually corrects itself within 24 hours; this can be initiated by stress, dehydration, and excessive alcohol intake.[1-3] As one gets older the tolerance for alcohol lessens, and even moderate amounts of drinking can lead to an episode of holiday heart.

Developing a balance between celebration and health can be a challenge. This article provides a brief overview of the literature on this topic, discusses causes of increased cardiac events during the holiday season, describes a patient profile and the effect on patients' health as well as on their families, and provides suggestions to decrease the risk of holiday heart during this festive time.

REVIEW OF LITERATURE

Ettinger and colleagues[1] conducted a study from 1972 to 1976, examining 32 separate dysrhythmic episodes requiring hospitalization in 24 patients who drank heavily before the onset of the arrhythmia. Patients were seen at 3 hospitals in New Jersey and were included in the study if they met the criteria of alcohol-associated arrhythmia, normal electrocardiogram (ECG) and chest radiograph, and no clinical evidence of heart disease. An association between excessive alcohol use and cardiac rhythm disorders is often difficult to establish in the absence of overt cardiomyopathy. None of the 24 patients had evidence of overt heart disease after treatment of arrhythmia. Episodes usually followed heavy drinking sprees at the weekend or on holiday, resulting in hospitalization between Sunday and Tuesday or in proximity to the year-end holidays. A relationship has not been observed in other alcohol-associated illnesses. Atrial fibrillation was the most common, but atrial flutter, tachycardia, junctional tachycardia, multiple atrial premature contractions, multiple premature ventricular contractions, and ventricular tachycardia were also observed. Transient hypokalemia was present with 4 of the 30 patients. Transient hypokalemia can cause a longer preejection period (PEP) and a shorter left ventricular ejection time (LVET). The mean PEP/LVET ratio after treatment was 0.412 ± 0.014 (normal 0.299 ± 0.008, $P<.0001$). High-speed, high-frequency recording of standard ECG limb leads were obtained at the same time. Heart rate, PR interval, QRS duration, and QT intervals were each measured and calculated in the 3 leads, and the longest duration of each was taken at the "true" duration. ECGs showed prolongation of PRc, QRS, and QTc. Typically these symptoms resolved rapidly, with spontaneous recovery with abstinence from alcohol use. This hallmark study coined the term "holiday heart syndrome."[2]

Phillips and colleagues[4] examined 53 million death certificates of cardiac and noncardiac deaths from 1973 to 2001 in the United States, and conducted a regression analysis of the daily estimated number of deaths expected during the holiday period. Given the null hypothesis, the number of deaths expected during the holiday period was then compared with the number of deaths observed. For noncardiac and cardiac mortalities, there was a spike in daily mortality occurring during the Christmas and New Year holiday period. This spike persisted after adjusting for trends and seasons, and was particularly large for individuals who were dead on arrival at a hospital, died in the emergency department (ED), or died as outpatients. For this group during the holiday period, 4.65% more cardiac and 4.99% more noncardiac deaths occurred than would be expected if the holidays did not affect mortality. Cardiac mortality for individuals who were dead on arrival, died in the ED, or died as outpatients peaked at Christmas and again at New Year. Multiple explanations for this association include, but are not limited to, delay in seeking treatment, respiratory diseases, emotional stresses associated with holidays, changes in diet and alcohol consumption, increased particulate pollution, month boundary effect, reporting artifact, postponement of death, and precipitation of death.[4]

Reedman and colleagues[5] conducted a retrospective analysis of a computerized billing database of ED visits. The study population consisted of a cohort of ED patients visiting 18 hospitals in New York and northern New Jersey from January 1, 1996 to November 30, 2004, analyzing HF patients from December 1 to January 31. The investigators compared the mean daily visits for the 2-week period of December 25 to January 7, as well as December 26 to December 30 and January 2 to January 5, using a Student t-test. The median age of patients was 77.3 years of age; women comprised 55.3% of the study population. Race demographics were not available from the database. The ratio of daily HF visits in December and January were compared with the mean daily HF visits in each month. The findings show a marked increase in the ratio of HF visits after Christmas and New Year's Day. Compared with other days of the months of December and January, there was a 23% (95% confidence interval, 14%–31%; $P<.001$) increase in the ratio of visits for December 25 to January 7. There was a marked increase in the 4-day period after the holidays; therefore, also reported was the ratio of the mean daily visits for the 4 days after Christmas to the mean for the rest of December and the 4 days after New Year's Day to the mean for the rest of January. There were significant findings during this period. There was a 33% and a 30% increase in the ratio of visits for HF mean daily visits after Christmas and New Year's Day, respectively. Every year was also separately analyzed. Each individual year showed variable increases in HF visits during the 2-week holiday period after Christmas and New Year's Day and in the 4 days after both Christmas and New Year's Day.[5]

Kloner and colleagues[6] analyzed 222,265 monthly death certificates from Los Angeles, California, for death caused by coronary artery disease from 1985 through 1996. The mean number of deaths was the highest in December, at 1808 and in January, at 1925; compared with the lowest rates in June, July, August, and September at 1402, 1424, 1418, and 1371, respectively. December and January had significantly higher rates than would be expected from a uniform distribution of monthly deaths. Monthly mortality correlated inversely with temperature. December and January were the months with the highest frequency of death, with an increase in deaths that peaked around the holiday season and then fell, which could not be explained solely on the basis of the daily temperature. Even in the mild climate of Los Angeles County, there are seasonal variations in death due to coronary artery disease, with approximately 33% more deaths occurring in December and January than in June through September. Although cooler temperatures may play a role, other factors such as overindulgence or stress of the holidays might also contribute to excess deaths during these peak times.[6]

Keatinge and Donaldson[7] conducted a study to see whether net mortalities increase during and after reeducation in medical services, either at average weekends or at Christmas, when pressure from illness is unusually high. Methods used were 2-fold paired t-test to compare mean daily deaths and hospital admissions during and after weekends (Saturday to Tuesday), with means for a week, in south-east England. The investigators also conducted linear regressions to see whether trends of daily deaths changed when admissions are reduced at Christmas. Deaths from all causes, respiratory, and ischemic heart disease were slightly reduced on Sundays by 1.6% and 2% when compared with the averages of the whole week. Ischemic heart mortality was also reduced on Saturdays to 1.9% below the whole-week averages. On Christmas Day, emergency admissions fell sharply below previous trends, and respiratory admissions fell by 18%. Respiratory deaths increased by 5.9% on December 26 and increased by 12.9% on December 27. No adverse effect on mortality was apparent within 2 days from reduction in medical services at weekends. However, respiratory deaths accelerated sharply after reduction in elective and emergency admissions at Christmas, when rates of infection and mortality from respiratory disease were high. That the increase in deaths after Christmas was confined to respiratory disease could be explained by the high level of respiratory infection at the time and by the fact that antibiotics, oxygen therapy, and positive-pressure ventilation can be life-saving in acute respiratory failure and can be most quickly given to patients who are already hospitalized.[7]

Barclay[8] outlines many adverse physical effects that have been related to alcohol consumption above recommended limits. In the cardiovascular system, all types of stroke have been associated with drinking, especially binge drinking. Alcohol use is a common cause of systolic and diastolic hypertension. It is long recognized that heavy alcohol consumption is the main cause of nonischemic, dilated cardiomyopathy. Heavy drinking increases the risk of cardiac arrhythmias regardless of the presence of heart disease. Atrial fibrillation is the best-known arrhythmia secondary to alcohol misuse, also known as holiday heart syndrome, but supraventricular and ventricular tachycardia also occur. Although alcohol has protective effects against coronary heart disease, at levels greater than 20 g alcohol will increase the risk.[8]

What is most important about this syndrome is that it usually occurs in someone with no known cardiac disease and may resolve when alcohol intake is ceased.[2] Patients with holiday heart syndrome can range in age from 30 to 70 years, and may or may not have a history of chronic alcohol use.[8] The type of alcohol is also insignificant in that holiday heart syndrome may occur just as often in those patients who drink wine and beer as in those who drink hard liquor.[8] One study found that as many as 66% of all new-onset atrial fibrillation cases in persons younger than 65 years were related to alcohol intoxication.[1] Although a variety of atrial and ventricular dysrhythmias have been associated with holiday heart syndrome, atrial fibrillation is most often seen, followed by atrial flutter and premature atrial and ventricular beat.[1,3,8,9] The exact mechanism of action for this alcohol-related dysrhythmia remains unclear. One theory is that alcohol or the metabolite of alcohol known as acetaldehyde may delay cardiac conduction times by facilitating the reentry phenomena.[3] Furthermore, acetaldehyde has been known to cause the release of myocardial norepinephrine, resulting in altered refractory periods and leaving the patient susceptible to tachycardic dysrhythmias such as atrial fibrillation, atrial flutter, and arterial and ventricular premature beats.[2,3] Honigman[9] posed another theory that alcohol itself decreases the fibrillation threshold, making the patient with alcohol intoxication more susceptible to dysrhythmias.

The main diagnostic sign of holiday heart syndrome is dysrhythmias. Other symptoms identified are palpitations, shortness of breath, chest pressure, atypical chest pain, syncope, and dizziness.[8-10] Laboratory evaluation is generally not helpful; cardiac markers should be evaluated to rule out acute myocardial infarction.[11] Blood alcohol levels are usually elevated and chest radiographs are usually normal.[11] Nonspecific ECG changes may be noted after the patient has converted to a normal sinus rhythm, such as absent septal Q, peaked or dimpled T waves, and PT prolongation, which will lead the practitioner to implicate alcohol in the disorder.[1-3,9,12]

CASE STUDY

C.G., a 20-year-old popular college student, is in her second year of her Bachelor of Nursing Program. She is excited to return home and spend the holidays with her parents and share some of her college moments with her younger sister. She was elected President of her sorority, chaired the social committee of her sorority, maintained a 3.5 grade point average and was on the junior varsity soccer team. She was relieved to have survived finals week and even more relieved that the sorority finals party, which lasted an entire weekend, was a huge success. She was drained and somewhat sad to say goodbye to her friends for the holidays, but she was thankful that the soccer team was on a break, as she felt more fatigued from this semester than the last.

Arriving home for the holidays, she is anxious to catch up with some hometown friends. Despite her exhaustion, she meets up with friends and they spend the night catching up over a few bottles of wine and good hometown pizza. The next morning C.G. skips her morning run, and complains of feeling fatigued and having some skipped heart beats. Her mother is concerned but attributes her daughter's symptoms to the hectic pace and the schedule she has kept over the last semester. Mother and daughter plan a Christmas shopping trip to the mall. While shopping, C.G. becomes short of breath walking in the mall and develops more palpitations, this time associated with chest pain.

Because of her nursing knowledge, C.G., in her mind, wonders if her potassium is too low: could she be having a heart attack at age 20? Or maybe her thyroid function is abnormal. "Oh, if only I would have paid more attention to that cardiology lecture," she thinks to herself. She does not feel well and at the insistence of her mother she makes an appointment to see her doctor. The doctor takes a detailed history. C.G. states she has no known allergies, is a nonsmoker, uses alcohol occasionally, and denies drug use. She describes being short of breath and fatigued since the end of finals week, with more palpitations and chest discomfort since last night. C.G. denies radiation of pain, has no syncope, and no rash. She drinks 3 caffeine beverages per day. Her only medication is birth-control pills that she has been on since age 17. Her family medical history is significant for myocardial infarction in her maternal and paternal grandfathers at age 70 and 75, respectively.

On physical examination C.G. looks fatigued but is awake and alert. She is afebrile, blood pressure 110/65, pulse irregular at a rate of 130 beats/min; oxygen saturation is 92% on room air but drops to 88% with minimal ambulation. Lung sounds have some crackles at the bases with moderate air exchange, abdomen is benign, and there is no edema in her lower extremities. A 12-lead ECG shows atrial fibrillation with rapid ventricular response. Her complete blood count, serum chemistries, and troponin level are all within normal ranges. Her blood alcohol level is elevated, at 94 mg/dL (normal 0–50 mg/dL).

C.G. is set up for a cardiac echocardiogram and is found to have normal ejection fraction and normal heart valves. She is diagnosed with holiday heart syndrome: she has some mild congestive HF caused by the atrial fibrillation with rapid ventricular response. She is given oral cardizem for control of heart rate, told to avoid alcohol, and is discharged from the observation unit 48 hours later. On follow-up visit the next week C.G. continues to be symptom-free and her ECG shows a normal sinus rhythm.

IMPLICATIONS

There are a few tactics that health care practitioners could consider for patients without established cardiac disease or with known risk factors for cardiac disease including, but not limited to[12]:

1. Instruct the patient to avoid delay in seeking medical attention, should cardiac symptoms occur.
2. Educate patients to maintain their medication schedule.
3. Educate patients to find time for physical activity. The American Heart Association recommends at least 30 minutes of moderate exercise most days of the week.
4. The importance of getting the flu shot: If the patient is older than 50 or has heart disease, getting the flu shot could help avoid influenza and protect against a heart attack or stroke.
5. Instruct the patient to take time and relax.
6. Educate the staff of the emergency departments and intensive care units to be aware of an increase in cardiac cases during the holiday season.
7. Educate patients to avoid known triggers
   a. Excess physical exertion (especially shoveling snow)
   b. Overeating
   c. Lack of sleep
   d. Emotional stress
   e. Illegal drugs
   f. Anger
   g. Excess salt and alcohol intake

SUMMARY

The increased number of deaths that occur from Thanksgiving to New Year's Day could be related to behavioral changes around the holiday season such as increased food, salt, and alcohol intake, and the way patients take their medications. The emotional and psychological stresses of the holidays may also contribute. Health care practitioners should be aware of holiday heart syndrome, and educate patients to help them minimize cardiac events during the holiday season. When evaluating patients during this season, clinicians should consider holiday-related factors and assess patients accordingly. Instead of adding or changing medications, patients should be reminded to follow their normal routines to minimize the risk of holiday heart and allow for more holiday enjoyment.

ACKNOWLEDGMENTS

The authors would like to thank Dr Arun Nagpaul, Medical Director at Newark Wayne Community Hospital, for providing the case scenario for this article.

REFERENCES

1. Ettinger PO, Wu CF, De la Cruz C, et al. Arrhythmias and the "holiday heart": alcohol associated cardiac rhythm disorders. Am Heart J 1978;95:555–62.
2. Sterner KL, Keough VA. Holiday heart syndrome: a case of cardiac irritability after increased alcohol consumption. J Emerg Nurs 2003;29:570–3.
3. Budzikowski A. Holiday heart syndrome—background. Available at: http://emedicine.medscape.com/article/155050-overview. Accessed February 23, 2012.

4. Phillips DP, Jarvinen JR, Abramson IS, et al. Cardiac mortality is higher around Christmas and New Year's than any other time: the holidays as a risk factor for death. Circulation 2004;100:3781–2.
5. Reedman LA, Allegra JR, Cochran DG. Increases in heart failure visits after Christmas and New Year's Day. Congest Heart Fail 2008;14:307–9.
6. Kloner RA, Poole WK, Perritt RL. When throughout the year is coronary death most likely to occur?: a 12 year population based analysis of more than 220,000 cases. Circulation 1999;100:1630–4.
7. Keatinge WR, Donaldson GC. Changes in mortalities and hospital admissions associated with holidays and respiratory illness: implications for medical services. J Eval Clin Pract 2005;11(3):275–81.
8. Barclay GA. Adverse physical effects of alcohol misuse. Adv Psychiatr Treat 2008;14:139–51.
9. Honigman B. Alcohol myopathy in cardiac and skeletal muscle. Top Emerg Med 1984;6:66–73.
10. Mittleman MA, Mostofsky E. Physical, psychological and chemical triggers of acute cardiovascular events. Preventive strategies. Circulation 2011;124:346–54.
11. Cotrell D. Atrial fibrillation: an emergency nurse's rapid response. J Emerg Nurs 2008;34:207–10.
12. Somes J, Donatelli NS. Syndromes of holiday heart. J Emerg Nurs 2012;37:577–9.

The Role of Vitamin D in Critical Illness

Zara R. Brenner, MS, RN-BC, ACNS-BC[a,b,*],
Arleen B. Miller, MS, APRN, CCRN[c], Lynn C. Ayers, MS, APRN, CCRN[d],
Ashlie Roberts, MS, APRN, CCRN[e,f]

KEYWORDS

- Critical illness • Vitamin D • Vitamin D deficiency

KEY POINTS

- Vitamin D deficiency has been linked to infectious processes and certain chronic disorders.
- Vitamin D deficiency present at the onset of critical illness may impact the severity of illness and contribute to less-than-optimal outcomes.
- The role of vitamin D supplementation in the critical care unit has not been established.

INTRODUCTION

The role of vitamin D as a beneficial nutrient in health and illness continues to be a controversial topic. As more research is conducted analyzing the effects of vitamin D, a lack of consensus still exists on the functions, appropriate levels, and usefulness in certain patient populations, including the critically ill.

Until recently, most health professionals thought that vitamin D deficiencies could be resolved with the fortification of milk and other food products. However, a comparison of 25-hydroxyvitamin D [25(OH)D] levels from the Third National Health and Nutrition Examination Survey (NHANES III) with NHANES 2001–2004 show that vitamin D levels in the United States are trending down.[1] People at risk for vitamin D deficiency are those who have less exposure to sunlight, who absorb less of the sun's rays, and

The authors have nothing to disclose.
[a] Care Management, Rochester General Hospital, 1425 Portland Avenue, Rochester, NY 14621, USA; [b] The College at Brockport, State University of New York, 350 New Campus Drive Brockport, NY 14420, USA; [c] 5800, Rochester General Hospital, 1425 Portland Avenue, Rochester, NY 14621, USA; [d] 4800, Rochester General Hospital, 1425 Portland Avenue, Rochester, NY 14621, USA; [e] Wegmans School of Nursing, St. John Fisher College, 3690 East Avenue, Rochester, NY 14618, USA; [f] Newark Wayne Community Hospital, PO Box 111 Driving Park Avenue, Newark, NY 14513, USA
* Corresponding author. Care Management, Rochester General Hospital, 1425 Portland Avenue, Rochester, NY 14621.
E-mail address: zararn@aol.com

who metabolize vitamin D less efficiently. See **Box 1** for a description of at-risk populations. Many of these risk factors are present in patients in intensive care units (ICUs). This article focuses on the physiology of vitamin D, the effects that deficiencies of vitamin D have on body systems, and the emerging role of vitamin D deficiency in critically ill patients.

PHYSIOLOGY OF VITAMIN D

Vitamin D is a steroid molecule that regulates the expression of many genes. Vitamin D, a fat-soluble vitamin, is found in 2 forms: vitamin D_2 (ergocalciferol) and vitamin D_3 (cholecalciferol). Ergocalciferol is found in yeast, fungi, and plants, but human intake is minimal. Cholecalciferol is made by the skin in response to as little as 15 minutes of ultraviolet (UV) irradiation each day and is also present in oil-rich fish, such as salmon. Vitamin D, whether ingested or resulting from UV exposure, is inert and must be activated by hydroxylation in the liver using cytochrome P450 enzymes. This reaction produces the circulating form, 25(OH)D or calciferol. 25(OH)D is further hydroxylated primarily in the proximal tubules of the kidney by the mitochondrial enzyme, 1 α-hydroxylase, into the active metabolite of vitamin D, 1,25-dihydroxy vitamin D [$1,25(OH)_2D$] or calcitriol. Although 25(OH)D has a half-life of several weeks, the half-life of $1,25(OH)_2D$ is limited to a few hours.

Vitamin D closely resembles a prohormone because its active form, $1,25(OH)_2D$, has characteristics more similar to those of a hormone than a vitamin. $1,25(OH)_2D$, principally a product of the kidney, circulates through the blood to exert its effects on target organs and tissues.[2,5] Regulation of $1,25(OH)_2D$ is controlled by a negative feedback loop whereby increased $1,25(OH)_2D$ stimulates parathyroid hormone to limit the production of circulating vitamin D.[6]

Because 25(OH)D has a longer half-life than $1,25(OH)_2D$, it is the more reliable laboratory marker.[3,5] Laboratory classification of vitamin D status is presented in **Table 1**. As a result of many studies, optimal vitamin D status today is best defined as a target serum 25(OH)D level of 75 nmol/L.[7]

Box 1
Populations at risk for vitamin D deficiency
People living in the very northern or very southern latitudes
People who are indoors in the winter
Darker-skinned people
The elderly
The obese
Exclusively breastfed infants
Vegans
Pregnant or lactating women
Postmenopausal women
Persons with chronic illness
Persons with fat malabsorption or lactose intolerance
Critically ill persons
Data from Refs.[2–4]

Table 1 Classification of vitamin D status by 25(OH)D concentration	
25(OH)D Concentration (ng/mL) (Hydroxyvitamin D)	Classification
≤10	Severe deficiency
10–20	Deficient
21–29	Insufficient
>30	Sufficient
75	Target serum level
>150	Toxicity

Data from Holick MF, Binkley NC, Bischoff-Ferrari HA, et al. Evaluation, treatment, and prevention of vitamin D deficiency: an endocrine society clinical practice guideline. J Clin Endocrinol Metab 2011;96:1911–30; and Hewison M. Antibacterial effects of vitamin D. Nat Rev Endocrinol 2011;7:337–5.

For a long time, vitamin D has been known for its role in optimizing neuromuscular and skeletal function. Vitamin D impacts intestinal absorption of calcium and phosphorus, renal excretion of phosphate, and bone resorption. Additionally, vitamin D receptors (VDRs) are situated in the nuclei of cells of multiple organs and the activation of these receptors results in an increased expression of more than 200 genes.[2] The activation of receptors in multiple genes is known as a pleiotropic effect.

Vitamin D has been shown to have an increasingly wide range of biologic functions, including inhibiting cellular proliferation, inhibiting angiogenesis (the growth of new blood vessels), stimulating insulin production, inhibiting renin production, and stimulating macrophage production of cathelicidin antimicrobial peptide (CAMP).[3] Vitamin D's newly recognized functions include action on macrophages, dendritic cells, lymphocytes, and epithelial cells, among others.[8]

THE CHALLENGES OF RESEARCHING THE ROLE OF VITAMIN D IN HUMAN ILLNESS

Research involving vitamin D in critical illness is a relatively new area of interest. There are significant challenges to establishing the impact of vitamin D deficiency on patients in the ICU. It is unknown if the vitamin D deficiency contributes to the development of the disease state or if the disease state contributes to the vitamin D deficiency. The influence of a third factor, known as confounding, may be a frequent occurrence. For example, a relationship between vitamin D deficiency and obesity may also be impacted by decreased exposure to sunlight. Studies can be limited by causality and by temporality (the impact of time).

Vitamin D and the Immune Response

As more research is conducted, explanations of vitamin D–dependent pathways in the immune system continue to develop. VDRs are found in various cells of the immune system, such as B lymphocytes, T lymphocytes, neutrophils, dendritic cells, monocytes, and macrophages.[9] Although predominantly a function of the renal tissue, the enzyme 1 α-hydroxylase is also expressed by tissues of the immune system. Consequently, cells from the immune system are capable of converting 25(OH)D into $1,25(OH)_2D$.[7]

Further evidence of the role of vitamin D as a direct inducer of antimicrobial innate immunity in humans is found in the Toll-like receptors (TLRs). The TLRs are part of the intracellular signaling that leads to proinflammatory cytokines as part of the immune response. TLRs recognize pathogens by their secretions as well as recognizing endogenous mediators released during inflammation. TLR activation in human monocytes and macrophages leads to an upregulation of VDR and vitamin-D-1 hydroxylase gene expression.[10] The upregulation of VDRs and vitamin-D-1 hydroxylase leads to increased expression of CAMP and the eventual secretion of CAMP in its active secretory form, LL-37. CAMP is active against a broad spectrum of infectious agents.[11] To prevent an overwhelming activation of TLRs, many innate substances modulate their expression and signaling.

Antimicrobial peptides are critical components of the immune response to bacterial, fugal, and viral infections. White and colleagues[12] screened VDR enzymes, identifying hundreds of 1,25(OH)$_2$D target genes. CAMP and B-defensin 4A (DEFB4A) are elements in 2 genes that encode antimicrobial peptides. CAMP expression is strongly stimulated by 1,25(OH)$_2$D in epithelial cells, macrophages/monocytes, and neutrophils. There is evidence to support that maintaining adequate vitamin D levels can protect against bacterial and viral pathogens.

Researchers have examined the association between vitamin D deficiency and infectious processes. Gombart's[6] review of the literature noted that vitamin D deficiency has been correlated with increased rates of respiratory infections, bacterial vaginosis in the first trimester of pregnancy, and accelerated progression of human immunodeficiency virus (HIV) in infected individuals. There have been suggestions that low levels of vitamin D can be associated with influenza epidemics and linked to an increased risk of and mortality rate from cancer. It has been proposed that replacing and maintaining vitamin D levels is beneficial for patients with multiple sclerosis, rheumatoid arthritis, diabetes, cardiovascular disease, and microbial infections.[6]

Although early studies demonstrated that exposure to UV rays treated tuberculosis, it is now suggested that it may be vitamin D, obtained from UV rays, that activates the monocytes that subsequently destroy the bacillus, *Mycobacterium tuberculosis*. Hewison[7] stated that 1,25(OH)$_2$D is unable to fight off *M tuberculosis* when RNA interference prevents the expression of either CAMP or DEFB4A. Because of the antibacterial and antiviral properties of CAMP, Hewison hypothesizes that vitamin D supplementation could have a broad range of innate immune activity.

The evidence is mounting for the function of vitamin D in regulating the immune system, specifically in response to viral infections.[13] Current research focuses on vitamin D and its role in fighting viral respiratory infections and the potential influence on HIV infections. Studies continue into the potential effect of vitamin D deficiency on the development of multiple sclerosis, hepatitis B and C, and dengue fever. The investigators concluded that current results support a hypothesis for vitamin D as an inhibitor of viruses.

VITAMIN D AND OBESITY

Obesity exerts a significant impact on the incidence of morbidity and mortality in the ICU. The Centers for Disease Control and Prevention classifies obesity as a body mass index (BMI) of greater than 30 kg/m^2 and estimates that greater than 33% of men and 35% of women fit into this category.[14] Low levels of vitamin D$_3$ have been linked to obesity in studies using BMI and waist circumference as markers. Confounders for lower levels of vitamin D in obese people include decreased physical activity, exposure to sunlight, vitamin D synthesis in subcutaneous fat, and/or sequestration in adipose tissue. However, it is unknown if a low vitamin D level is a contributor to the development of obesity.[15]

When obese and nonobese adults received vitamin D replacement therapy, either by sunlight (UV) or oral supplementation, obese adults were only able to raise their vitamin D serum levels by 50% in comparison with nonobese adults.[3] Obese adults are at greater risk for vitamin D deficiency as a result of sequestration of vitamin D in the adipose tissue. Thus, a vitamin D deficiency may lead to secondary hyperparathyroidism because of the decreased bioavailability of vitamin D.

Lira and colleagues[16] examined the effects of supplementing vitamins D and E on the levels of interleukin (IL)-6 and IL-10 protein expression in the adipose tissue of mice provided with a high-fat diet (HFD). IL-6 is considered a major inflammatory mediator in obesity, having been implicated in the release of triglycerides and free fatty acids, downregulated lipoprotein lipase, insulin resistance, increased production of reactive oxygen species, and decreased nitric oxide generation. IL-10 may antagonize the effects of IL-6. After 30 days of treatment with vitamin D_3 and vitamin E, the mice receiving an HFD with vitamins E and D_3 supplementation compared with the HFD alone showed a significant decrease in body weight gain ($P<.001$). The IL-6 level in adipose tissue was decreased ($P = .05$) as was the IL-6/IL-10 ratio ($P = .01$) in the group's vitamins D and E supplements. These researchers hypothesized that, for adults, vitamin D and E supplements could be used as adjunctive therapy to reduce proinflammatory cytokine levels in obese patients.

An inverse relationship has been found between vitamin D_3 levels and HbA1c whereby HbA1c serves as a marker for type II diabetes in obese adults (BMI levels 28–50 kg/m^2). An inverse relationship was also demonstrated for the correlation between vitamin D_3 levels and each of the following measurements: body weight, BMI, and waist circumference.[17] However, researchers were unable to establish relationships between vitamin D levels and the mass of adipose tissue and/or metabolic syndrome.

Lee and Campbell[15] reviewed correlational research with vitamin D and obesity and found multiple outcomes. Ionized parathyroid hormone (PTH) levels were higher in obese young adults as compared with nonobese young adults. As obese patients lost weight, their PTH decreased. Secondary hyperparathyroidism can result from vitamin D deficiency and lead to a compensatory increase in 1,25 (OH)$_2$D. Additionally, increased PTH levels can increase calcium concentration in adipose tissue, which can lead to an increase in lipids.

Parathyroid hormone level was an independent predictor of metabolic syndrome, as characterized by abdominal obesity, insulin resistance, dyslipidemia, hyperglycemia, and hypertension, in a group of 1017 morbidly obese Caucasian patients.[18] However, magnesium and 25(OH)D levels were not significant in predicting metabolic syndrome.

THE ROLE OF VITAMIN D IN CARDIOVASCULAR FUNCTION

In critically ill patients, vitamin D deficiency has been associated with myocardial infarction and cardiac failure. There is increasing evidence to suggest that low vitamin D levels contribute to cardiovascular disease states, such as left ventricular hypertrophy, hypertension, coronary artery calcification, myocardial infarction, heart failure, endothelial dysfunction, and stroke.[19] Vitamin D is thought to affect several mechanisms in cardiovascular function. The renin-angiotensin-aldosterone system (RAAS) is key to controlling blood pressure. The vascular response to stress includes arterial stiffness, which can progress to cardiovascular disease. VDRs are present in the endothelial cells and are upregulated when the body is under stress. Thus, vitamin D acts to suppress the RAAS and improve endothelium function. Furthermore, the role of vitamin D in regulating lymphocytes and monocytes and limiting the release of inflammatory cytokines can increase the retention of cholesterol in the vascular walls.[20] In addition, vitamin D deficiency causes secondary hyperparathyroidism, which could accelerate its harmful effects on the cardiovascular system. Low vitamin D levels decrease absorption of calcium in the intestines causing the release of PTH. Increased PTH levels lead to an increase in blood pressure and myocardial contractility, which can contribute to left ventricular hypertrophy and vascular remodeling.[21]

Wang and colleagues[22] used a prospective review of 1739 Framingham Offspring Study participants to study the effects of low vitamin D levels on the cardiovascular system. The study included a physician-administered medical history, examination, and laboratory assessment. Analysis revealed an increase in coronary heart disease and hypertension in regions of the world with less exposure to sunlight. Prior studies did not include other mineral markers, such as phosphorus and calcium, which also have plaque-producing qualities. The mechanism by which low vitamin D levels affects the cardiovascular health of an individual remains unclear.

Sun and colleagues[23] conducted a prospective research study consisting of 74 272 women and 44 592 men in the United States with a predominant European ancestry using The Nurses' Health Study for female nurses and the Health Professionals Follow-up Study for male health professionals. The population had no prior evidence of cardiovascular disease or cancer. Data suggested an association between a higher intake of vitamin D and a lower risk of cardiovascular disease in men but not in women. This finding could be related to vitamin D levels too low to produce any meaningful difference and/or to the tendency of women to have a higher percentage of body fat than men. The investigators suggested that it may be useful to study estrogen levels in women and whether replacement of these low levels after menopause would have a positive or negative effect on this evidence.

There are no data available to suggest the appropriate vitamin D levels needed to support cardiovascular health.[24] Few studies have evaluated the effect of vitamin D replacement on cardiovascular outcomes; the results have been inconclusive or contradictory.[19] More studies are needed to determine the role of vitamin D in cardiovascular disease.

THE ROLE OF VITAMIN D IN LUNG FUNCTION

Critically ill patients develop decreased lung function from multiple pathologies. An analysis of data collected for NHANES III to explore pulmonary indicators found that there was a strong relationship between serum concentrations of 25(OH)D, forced expiratory volume in the first second of expiration, and forced vital capacity.[25] Several lung diseases, all inflammatory in nature, may be related to activities of vitamin D, including asthma, chronic obstructive pulmonary disease (COPD), and cancer. However, it is not known whether there is a causal relationship between acute respiratory distress, lung injury, and vitamin D deficiency.

The role of vitamin D in mediating acute pulmonary inflammatory diseases and how this relationship might impact critically ill patients remains unclear. Vitamin D impacts inflammatory and structural cells, including dendritic cells, lymphocytes, monocytes, and epithelial cells. Calcitriol inhibits the formation of matrix metalloproteinases, which play an important role in tissue remodeling, and those tissue changes are thought to be significant in respiratory disease. In addition, calcitriol inhibits fibroblast proliferation and influences collagen synthesis, both of which are significant events in normal tissue repair and in fibrotic lesion formation.[8]

A review of the literature examined correlations between vitamin D and lung diseases, including COPD, asthma, cystic fibrosis, and interstitial pneumonia.[26] They concluded that there was strong evidence to show a relationship between vitamin D deficiency and chronic lung disease, especially COPD and asthma. The relationship between pulmonary decompensation that requires mechanical ventilation and vitamin D deficiency was less clear. The investigators recommended further studies to explore any direct effects of vitamin D on the mechanisms of lung injury and lung function.

Hansdottir and Monick[27] completed a recent review of the literature regarding the effects of vitamin D on lung immunity and respiratory diseases. The investigators stated that epidemiologic studies suggest an association between low vitamin D levels and mycobacterial infections, respiratory viral infections, and asthma. The connection may be related, in part, to the expression of 1 α-hydroxylase by airway epithelium, macrophages, dendritic cells, and lymphocytes in the respiratory tract, thus, indicating that active vitamin D may be produced locally within the lungs. The investigators concluded that mechanistic questions remain and clinical trials are needed.

Zosky and colleagues[28] explored the in vivo effect of vitamin D deficiencies on lung structure and function. Using a vitamin D–deficient multigenerational mouse model, the authors examined lung volume, mechanics, and structure. They concluded that in mice there was a direct role of vitamin D in a causal relationship with decreased lung function.

VITAMIN D AND BONE TURNOVER IN THE INTENSIVE CARE UNIT (ICU)

The relationship between bone health and vitamin D deficiency is well established. In adults, osteomalacia is used to describe bone disease caused by vitamin D deficiency. Proximal muscle weakness and gait instability are associated with osteomalacia, causing an increased risk of falls and fractures, which are concerns for all nurses in every ICU.[5,29]

Vitamin D has a role in maintaining serum calcium levels and, therefore, bone health through a direct effect on calcium absorption and excretion through a series of inter-relationships with serum phosphate and parathyroid hormone in the PTH–vitamin D axis.[4,30] Hypocalcemia is prevented by 3 mechanisms, one of which is the release of calcium from the skeleton through bone resorption mediated by 1,25(OH)$_2$D.[30]

Many patients have compromised levels of vitamin D before entering the ICU. Critically ill patients on prolonged bed rest are at a greater risk of bone loss and osteoporosis. Recovery from bone loss associated with a prolonged vitamin D deficiency can be very difficult. In addition, people who are vitamin D deficient absorb smaller amounts of phosphorous and even smaller amounts of calcium in the intestine. Hypocalcemia, which is frequently seen in critically ill patients, causes an increase in parathyroid simulation. Parathyroid hormone stimulates the tubular reabsorption of calcium, which stimulates the kidneys to produce 1, 25(OH)$_2$D, and is responsible for the activation of osteoblasts. When activated, osteoblasts stimulate the transformation of preosteoclasts into mature osteoclasts. The mature osteoclasts are responsible for the demineralization of bone seen in osteoporosis.[3]

In a study conducted by Van den Berghe and colleagues,[31] prolonged critical illness was defined as patients requiring full organ support, including mechanical ventilation for greater than 7 days. The investigators concluded that severe bone hyper-resorption and compromised osteoblast function were associated with extended time in the ICU. Furthermore, the typically recommended daily supplementation of vitamin D did not meet the needs of critically ill patients. The investigators stated that further studies are needed to understand the increased bone turnover observed in these patients to prevent any long-term consequences.

VITAMIN D IN SEPSIS

Sepsis is a too-frequent occurrence in critically ill patients. Despite the creation of the sepsis bundle and a national program to decrease the occurrence of sepsis in hospitalized patients, it remains a problem. The role of vitamin D in the inflammatory response remains unclear and researchers continue to explore the function of vitamin D in sepsis.

Lee and Campbell[15] proposed a hypothetical model that links a low level metabolic endotoxemia in the gut, regulated in part by lipopolysaccharide (LPS), an endotoxin, and a vitamin D–deficient decreased immune response. The combination of metabolic endotoxemia and vitamin D deficiency becomes a synergistic reaction in obese patients. The investigators suggested that low-grade inflammation in obese individuals is enhanced as macrophages migrate from the vitamin D–insufficient systemic circulation into the adipose tissue.

The UV Foundation, the Vitamin D Society, and the European Sunlight Association funded an epidemiologic review of the literature.[32] Septicemia rates were noted to be higher in the winter than in the fall, highest in the Northeast United States and lowest in the West, higher for African Americans and other people of color, increased with age, higher in men, and higher in urban areas. Those with a higher BMI have an increased risk for death. Because many of these descriptive categories are also identified in those individuals with lower vitamin D levels, the investigator proposed that the impact of higher levels of 25(OH)D on the incidence and prognosis of septicemia "should be easy to test."[32] Nonetheless, research about the role of vitamin D in critically ill human patients with sepsis is limited.

Animal studies have shown that the administration of 25(OH)D improved coagulation in sepsis-associated disseminated intravascular coagulation; modulated inflammatory cytokines, such as TNF-α and IL-6; as well as inhibited LPS-induced vasodilation of the vascular endothelium. Research has found enhanced expression of LL-37, the endogenous antimicrobial peptide, at barrier sites, including respiratory and colonic epithelium, saliva, and skin. Jeng and colleagues[11] examined the plasma levels of 25(OH)D, vitamin D–binding protein, and LL-37 in 3 groups of patients. The researchers measured levels in 24 ICU patients with sepsis, 25 ICU patients who did not have sepsis, and 21 healthy controls. Their findings demonstrated that although vitamin D deficiency was highly prevalent in all 3 populations, critically ill patients had lower levels of 25(OH)D than healthy controls, even after adjusting for race. They also found that vitamin D–binding protein levels were significantly lower in critically ill patients with sepsis compared with both other groups. In addition, the researchers showed that lower levels of 25(OH)D were associated with lower levels of LL-37.

A retrospective study of ICU patients admitted with sepsis (n = 92) and those admitted with trauma (n = 72) found differences in median vitamin D levels.[33] Patients with criteria often correlated with low vitamin D levels, such as age less than 18 years, malnutrition, pregnancy or lactation, malignancies, pathologies affecting bone and calcium metabolism, and those undergoing immunotherapy, were excluded from the study. The median vitamin D level in the sepsis group was 10.1 ng/mL, whereas the trauma group had a median vitamin D level of 18.4 ng/mL (P<.0001). Patients with sepsis showed a significantly higher procalcitonin level (P<.0001) on admission to the ICU. There was no significant difference in length of stay between the two groups; although the mortality rate was higher in the sick patients with sepsis (27.9% vs 11.1% in the healthy trauma patients), that rate was also not significant.

Vitamin D levels were obtained from 81 patients identified as having infection without sepsis (n = 16), with sepsis (n = 22), or severe sepsis (n = 43) on admission to the emergency department and again 24 hours later.[34] Vitamin D insufficiency was associated with all markers of illness at both time points, including severe sepsis, elevated Acute Physiology Age Chronic Health Evaluation (APACHE) II scores, and higher Sepsis-related Organ Failure Assessment scores. Additionally, all 4 patients who died during the hospitalization had 25(OH)D levels of less than 75 nmol/L.

MORBIDITY AND MORTALITY AND VITAMIN D

Vitamin D deficiency is known to be associated with disease states in the general population. There are numerous manifestations of vitamin D deficiency in the general population and in chronic illnesses. Vitamin D deficiency present at the onset of critical illness may relate to the severity of illness and contribute to less-than-optimal outcomes. Unfortunately, high mortality and critical illness have a symbiotic relationship. Vitamin D insufficiency has been associated with a greater incidence of many pathologic states that affect mortality, whereas higher vitamin D levels are associated with a decreased incidence of and adverse outcomes from hypertension, diabetes mellitus, cardiovascular disease, cancer, and infection. Because of these associations, studies are underway that examine the intricacies of critical illness, vitamin D, and how or what can be done to decrease morbidity and mortality.

Lee and colleageus[35] estimated that 50% of ICU patients are either vitamin D insufficient or deficient, with 17% of the critically ill patients having undetectable levels of vitamin D. The investigators explored the pathways by which a vitamin D–deficient state contributes to the deterioration of the existing immune response and other multiple metabolic dysfunctions in the critically ill population, leading to poorer patient outcomes (**Fig. 1**). They noted that 1 α-hydroxylase, the enzyme that converts 25(OH)D into $1,25(OH)_2D$, although found in larger amounts in the kidney, is also found in almost all human cells. This concept explains why hypocalcemia and hypoparathyroidism, which are both markers of vitamin D deficiency, relate to disease severity. It also explains why calcium replacement has not been shown to improve outcomes.

Grant and colleagues[36] conducted a meta-analysis with an emphasis on Canadians. They performed a literature search for dose-response relationships for vitamin D indices and disease outcomes using 2005 mortality data from Statistics Canada. The investigators estimated that the death rate in Canada could be reduced by 16.1% if the mean serum 25(OH)D level was increased from 67 to 105 nmol/L. Heart disease deaths would decrease by 12.9%, and cancer deaths would decrease by 16.8%.

A cross-sectional study by McKinney and colleagues[37] found that low levels of vitamin D were linked to adverse and more costly outcomes in relation to *Clostridium difficile* and methicillin-resistant *Staphylococcus aureus* infections. The investigators reported that low albumin levels were associated with low vitamin D status and, as such, could be considered a confounding variable. Nonetheless, patients with low levels of vitamin D had a greater length of stay and an increase in the number of repeat hospitalizations.

Older adults, who constitute a large segment of critically ill patients, are at high risk for vitamin D insufficiency. A prospective observational study by Ginde and colleagues[1] was conducted with 3408 NHANES III participants aged 65 years and older. The results demonstrated that the baseline 25(OH)D values were inversely associated with all-cause mortality (adjusted hazard ratio, 0.95; 95% confidence interval, 0.92–0.98) per 10 nmol/L 25(OH)D. The association seemed stronger for cardiovascular disease (CVD) mortality than for non-CVD mortality (adjusted hazard ratio, 2.36; 95% confidence interval, 1.17–4.75). The investigators also reported an apparent dose-response association with the largest risk in the lowest 25(OH)D stratum (<25.0 nmol/L) (adjusted hazard ratio, 1.83; 95% confidence interval, 1.14–2.94). The association between 25(OH)D and all-cause mortality was stronger in those with diabetes mellitus at baseline than those without (adjusted hazard ratios, 0.86 and 0.96, respectively; $P = .02$ [for interaction]). The investigators concluded that based on all-cause mortality, current dosage recommendations for vitamin D supplementation in noninstitutionalized individuals seems to be inadequate.

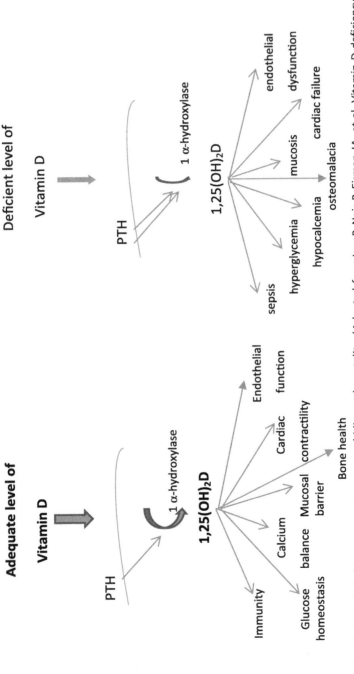

Fig. 1. Vitamin D in clinical improvement versus morbidity and mortality. (*Adapted from* Lee P, Nair P, Eisman JA, et al. Vitamin D deficiency in the intensive care unit: an invisible accomplice to morbidity and mortality. Intensive Care Med 2009;35:2028–32; with permission.)

VITAMIN D SUPPLEMENTS IN THE ICU?

There are emerging links between vitamin D levels, decreased mortality, and better patient outcomes. Yet there is currently insufficient evidence to recommend the use of vitamin D dosing in the ICU. Defining a vitamin D level at which therapeutic supplementation for critically ill patients should occur is complex for many reasons. Optimal levels are changing as the low end of normal is being raised. There is wide individual variability in vitamin D interaction with calcium intake.[5] The ideal level of vitamin D needed for prevention versus treatment of disease may be different. The level needed to prevent osteomalacia is different from the level at which parathyroid hormone suppression occurs, which is also different from the level at which intestinal calcium absorption is optimized.[28] Effective vitamin D supplementation may be different for critically ill patients compared with other individuals.

Lee and colleagues[30] suggest that vitamin D deficiency is an "invisible accomplice to morbidity and mortality" in critically ill patients. The impact of vitamin D deficiency in chronic illness has been described, yet the impact of that same vitamin D deficiency in critically ill patients has not been fully explored (**Table 2**). Vitamin D deficiency "may worsen existing organ dysfunctions in critically ill patients, leading to worse outcomes." Within the concept of critical illness, they propose that the "potential for vitamin D therapy is important" because it is inexpensive and has a wide therapeutic window.

As vitamin D deficiency becomes more closely associated with poorer outcomes, the following question must be asked: should we be giving vitamin D supplements to critically ill patients? Researchers are beginning to determine the efficacy and effectiveness of vitamin D supplementation in the outcomes of critically ill patients.[38,39]

Amrein and colleagues[39] conducted a small, randomized double-blind placebo-controlled pilot study to evaluate the safety and efficacy of a single high dose of

Table 2
Potential manifestations among critically ill patients of known association of vitamin D deficiency seen in the general population

Known Functions of Vitamin D	Known Association in General Population	Potential Manifestations of Association in Critically Ill Patients
Cardiovascular function	Atherosclerosis, hypertension, myocardial infarction, cardiac failure	Impaired microcirculation, organ failure, cardiogenic shock
Neuronal/cognitive function	Stroke, Alzheimer disease, diabetic neuropathy	Coma, slow neurologic recovery, critical illness polyneuropathy
Glucose metabolism	Diabetes	Hyperglycemia
Bone turnover, calcium homeostasis	Osteomalacia, osteoporosis	Hypocalcemia, hypoparathyroidism, fractures
Lung function	Chronic obstructive pulmonary disease	Acute lung injury, respiratory failure
Immune system	Tuberculosis, autoimmune diseases, inflammatory bowel disease, neoplasms	Nosocomial infections, mucositis, translocation of bowel flora, systemic inflammatory response syndrome, sepsis
Muscle function	Myopathy, myalgia	Critical illness myopathy, falls

Adapted from Lee P, Nair P, Eisman JA, et al. Vitamin D deficiency in the intensive care unit: an invisible accomplice to morbidity and mortality. Intensive Care Med 2009;35:2028–32.

oral vitamin D in critically ill, vitamin D–deficient patients in a medical ICU. Twenty-five patients with vitamin D levels less than 20 ng/mL and who were expected to have an ICU stay greater than 48 hours were divided into 2 groups. The experimental group (n = 12) received 540,000 IU vitamin D dissolved in an herbal oil either orally or via a feeding tube. The control group (n = 13) received a placebo. The groups were similar in baseline characteristics. The mean serum 25(OH)D increase in the intervention group was 25 ng/dL. Both total serum calcium ($P<.05$) and total ionized calcium ($P<.05$) increased in the treatment group. Hypercalcemia and hypercalciuria did not occur in any patient. Changes in parathyroid hormone levels between the two groups were not significant. There were no differences in clinical outcomes, including duration of mechanical ventilation, duration of vasopressor therapy, length of stay after initiation of the study, ICU days after initiation of the study, or mortality. The investigators stated that no adverse effects were observed in response to the single high dose of oral vitamin D and that the single dose was effective in raising vitamin D levels.

Flynn and colleagues[40] prospectively examined the effects of vitamin D deficiency in critically ill surgical patients. The 49 patients (74%) admitted with 25(OH)D levels less than 20 ng/mL had longer hospital stays than the 17 patients with vitamin D levels of 20 ng/mL or more ($P = .03$). Patients with 25(OH)D levels less than 20 ng/mL tended to have longer ICU stays ($P = .3$), higher rates of infection ($P = .09$), and a higher incidence of sepsis ($P = .29$). There were no differences in mortality. The investigators reported that 21 patients with 25(OH)D levels less than 20 ng/mL and APACHE II scores of 18 or more compared with patients with 25(OH)D levels of 20 ng/mL or more and the same APACHE II scores had a longer hospital stay ($P <.0001$), longer ICU stay ($P<.001$), and a higher rate of infection ($P = .005$). Vitamin D supplements were given to patients who were able to receive oral medications (n = 33). Of those patients who had more than one vitamin D level determined, only 11 had significant improvement in their vitamin D level over the course of their hospital stay. The investigators concluded that vitamin D levels less than 20 ng/mL have a significant impact on length of stay, organ dysfunction, and infection rates and that more data are needed on the value of supplementation to improve patient outcomes.

SUMMARY

The role of vitamin D in multiple body systems, disease states, infectious processes, and critical illness is becoming increasingly evident. Although vitamin D deficiency present at the onset of critical illness may relate to the severity of illness and contribute to poorer patient outcomes, there is not enough evidence to support adding vitamin D assessment to routine intensive care workload or costs. Some recent data suggest that vitamin D deficiency may prolong hospital stays and increase patients' risk of infection, but the role for vitamin D supplementation in the ICU has yet to be established. As health care team members develop an increased awareness of the potential benefits of normalized vitamin D levels, there will be an increased interdisciplinary discussion regarding measurement and supplementation. Nurses will be involved in clinical research trials being conducted to confirm the promise of vitamin D in the therapy of critically ill patients.

REFERENCES

1. Ginde AA, Scragg R, Schwartz RS, et al. Prospective study of serum 25-hydroxyvitamin D, cardiovascular disease mortality and all-cause mortality in older US adults. J Am Geriatr Soc 2009;57:1595–603.

2. Bell DS. Protean manifestations of vitamin D deficiency, part 1: the epidemic of deficiency. South Med J 2011;104:331–4.
3. Holick MF, Binkley NC, Bischoff-Ferrari HA, et al. Evaluation, treatment, and prevention of vitamin D deficiency: an endocrine society clinical practice guideline. J Clin Endocrinol Metab 2011;96:1911–30.
4. Cannell JJ, Hollis BW, Zasloff M, et al. Diagnosis and treatment of vitamin D deficiency. Expert Opin Pharmacother 2008;9:107–18.
5. Thacher TD, Clarke BL. Vitamin D insufficiency. Mayo Clin Proc 2011;86:50–60.
6. Gombart A. The vitamin D-antimicrobial peptide pathway and its role in protection against infection. Future Microbiol 2009;4:1151–65.
7. Hewison M. Antibacterial effects of vitamin D. Nat Rev Endocrinol 2011;7:337–45.
8. Herr C, Greulich T, Koczulla RA, et al. The role of vitamin D in pulmonary disease: COPD, asthma, infection, and cancer. Respir Res 2011;12:31.
9. Di Rosa M, Malaguarnera M, Nicoletti F, et al. Vitamin D3: a helpful immuno-modulator. Immunology 2011;134:123–39.
10. Wittebole X, Castanares-Zapatero D, Laterre PF. Toll-like receptor 4 modulation as a strategy to treat sepsis. Mediators Inflamm 2010;2010:568396.
11. Jeng L, Yamshchikov AV, Judd SE, et al. Alterations in vitamin D status and antimicrobial peptide levels in patients in the intensive care unit with sepsis. J Transl Med 2009;7:28–37.
12. White JH. Vitamin D as an inducer of cathelicidin antimicrobial peptide expression: past, present and future. J Steroid Biochem Mol Biol 2010;121:234–8.
13. Beard JA, Bearden A, Striker R. Vitamin D and the anti-viral state. J Clin Virol 2011;50:194–200.
14. Flegal K, Carroll M, Ogden C, et al. Prevalence and trends in obesity among US adults, 1999–2008. JAMA 2010;303:235–41.
15. Lee P, Campbell LV. Vitamin D deficiency: the invisible accomplice of metabolic endotoxemia? Curr Pharm Des 2009;15:2751–8.
16. Lira FS, Rosa JC, Cunha CA, et al. Supplementing alpha-tocopherol (vitamin E) and vitamin D3 in high fat diet decrease IL-6 production in murine epididymal adipose tissue and 3T3-L1 adipocytes following LPS stimulation. Lipids Health Dis 2011;10:37.
17. McGill A, Stewart J, Lithander F, et al. Relationships of low serum vitamin D3 with anthropometry and markers of the metabolic syndrome and diabetes in overweight and obesity. Nutr J 2008;7:4.
18. Hjelmesaeth J, Hofso D, Aasheim E, et al. Parathyroid hormone, but not vitamin D, is associated with the metabolic syndrome in morbidly obese women and men: a cross-sectional study. Cardiovasc Diabetol 2009;8:7.
19. McGreevey C, Williams D. New insights about vitamin D and cardiovascular disease. Ann Intern Med 2011;155:820–6.
20. Al Mheid I, Patel R, Murrow, et al. Vitamin D status is associated with arterial stiffness and vascular dysfunction in healthy humans. J Am Coll Cardiol 2011;58(2):186–92.
21. Sarkinen B. Vitamin D deficiency & cardiovascular disease. Nurse Pract 2011;36:46–53.
22. Wang TJ, Pencina MJ, Booth SL, et al. Vitamin D deficiency and risk of cardiovascular disease. Circulation 2008;117:503–11.
23. Sun Q, Shi L, Rimm EB, et al. Vitamin D intake and risk of cardiovascular disease in US men and women. Am J Clin Nutr 2011;94:534–42.
24. Carrelli AL, Walker MD, Lowe H, et al. Vitamin d deficiency is associated with subclinical carotid atherosclerosis: the northern Manhattan study. Stroke 2011;42(8):2240–5.

25. Black PN, Scragg R. Relationship between serum 25-hydroxyvitamin D and pulmonary function in the third national health and nutrition examination survey. Chest 2005;128:3792–8.
26. Gilbert CR, Arum SM, Smith CM. Vitamin D deficiency and chronic lung disease. Can Respir J 2009;16:75–80.
27. Hansdottir S, Monick MM. Vitamin D effects on lung immunity and respiratory diseases. Vitam Horm 2011;86:217–37.
28. Zosky GR, Berry LJ, Elliot JG, et al. Vitamin D deficiency causes deficits in lung function and alters lung structure. Am J Respir Crit Care Med 2011;183:1336–43.
29. Holick MF. Vitamin D deficiency. N Engl J Med 2007;357:266–81.
30. Lee P, Nair P, Eisman JA, et al. Vitamin D deficiency in the intensive care unit: an invisible accomplice to morbidity and mortality. Intensive Care Med 2009;35:2028–32.
31. Van Den Berghe G, Van Roosbroeck D, Vanhove P, et al. Bone turnover in prolonged critical illness: effect of vitamin D. J Clin Endocrinol Metab 2003;88:4623–32.
32. Grant WB. Solar ultraviolet-B irradiance and vitamin D may reduce the risk of septicemia. Dermatoendocrinol 2009;1:37–42.
33. Cecchi A, Bonizzoli M, Douar S, et al. Vitamin D deficiency in septic patients at ICU admission is not a mortality predictor. Minerva Anestesiol 2011;77:1184–9.
34. Ginde AA, Camargo CA Jr, Shapiro NI. Vitamin D insufficiency and sepsis severity in emergency department patients with suspected infection. Acad Emerg Med 2009;18:551–4.
35. Lee P, Eisman JA, Center JR. Vitamin D deficiency in critically ill patients. N Engl J Med 2009;360:1912–4.
36. Grant WB, Schwalfenberg GK, Genuis SJ, et al. An estimate of the economic burden and premature deaths due to vitamin D deficiency in Canada. Mol Nutr Food Res 2010;54:1172–81.
37. McKinney JD, Bailey BA, Garrett LH, et al. Relationship between vitamin D status and ICU outcomes in veterans. J Am Med Dir Assoc 2011;12:208–11.
38. Higgins D. Impact of vitamin D deficiency on outcomes in critically ill patients. JPEN J Parenter Enteral Nutr 2011;35:134.
39. Amrein K, Sourij H, Wagner G, et al. Short-term effects of high dose oral vitamin D in critically ill vitamin D deficient patients: a randomized double blind, placebo controlled pilot study. Crit Care 2011;15(2):R104.
40. Flynn L, Zimmerman LH, McNorton K, et al. Effects of vitamin deficiency in critically ill surgical patients. Am J Surg 2011. http://dx.doi.org/10.1016/amjsurg.2011.09.012.

Viral Gastroenteritis in the Adult Population: The GI Peril

Maureen E. Krenzer, MS, RN, ACNS-BC

KEYWORDS

- Gastroenteritis • Gastrointestinal illness • Adult • Elderly • Rehydration • Norovirus
- Vomiting • Diarrhea

KEY POINTS

- Viral gastroenteritis is common and causes diarrhea in all age groups worldwide.
- Norovirus is the leading cause of viral gastroenteritis for adults.
- Norovirus is a winter peril because of the combination of low infectious dose, viral shedding for a long duration before and after illness, and resistance with low temperatures.
- Dehydration and hypovolemia are consequences for complicated cases of gastroenteritis in vulnerable populations.

INTRODUCTION

Acute infectious diarrhea is caused by viruses, bacteria, and protozoa. In mild cases patients may not even contact their health care provider, and even if they do, stools may not be tested. A careful history should include the duration of symptoms and the frequency and characteristics of stool. Severe diarrhea alone, defined as greater than 4 liquid stools per day for more than 3 days, is often a bacterial cause. Fever and peritoneal signs may indicate infection with an enteric pathogen. Blood in the stool is usually an indication of an inflammatory process from invasive bacteria. Residence, recent and remote travel, occupational exposures, pets, and hobbies can provide clues to the origin of the diarrhea. Studies have shown that most cases of acute infectious gastroenteritis are viral. This article focuses on viral gastroenteritis.

Viral gastroenteritis is inflammation of the lining of the stomach, small intestine, and large intestine. Viral gastroenteritis is extremely common and causes millions of cases of diarrhea annually.[1] This disease affects infants, adults, and the elderly population alike and is a worldwide issue and major public health concern. The financial burden to society through direct and indirect costs can be overwhelming. The death rate worldwide continues to be high but has improved over recent decades because of early treatment, including use of oral rehydration therapy and improved nutrition

The author has nothing to disclose.
Department of Nursing, Rochester General Hospital, 1425 Portland Avenue, Rochester, NY 14621, USA
E-mail address: maureen.krenzer@rochestergeneral.org

and water sanitation measures. Most people recover completely without any complications as long as they avoid dehydration.

TYPES OF VIRUSES

The 4 major groups of viruses that cause viral gastroenteritis are Caliciviridae (primarily norovirus), enteric adenoviruses, astrovirus, and rotavirus. Other infrequent causes of gastroenteritis include bocaviruses, coronaviruses, toroviruses, Aichi virus, picobirnavirus, and cytomegalovirus.[2] The "stomach flu" is not viral gastroenteritis because it is not caused by the influenza virus.

Norovirus, also called *Norwalk-like viruses*, named after the location in which the first outbreak was identified, is a single positive-strand RNA virus with a nonenveloped protein coat and cup-shaped depression.[2] This group of viruses includes many genotypes and subgroups, likely because of mutations developed during RNA replications. The GII.4 strain has evolved as the pandemic strain in the United States.[2] Norovirus can be seen throughout the year but predominantly between November and April. It can affect patients of all ages. Norovirus is recognized as the leading cause of foodborne-disease outbreaks in the United States. The Centers for Disease Control and Prevention (CDC) estimates that each year more than 20 million cases of acute gastroenteritis are caused by noroviruses.[3]

Sapovirus is another virus in the Calciviridae family that can affect children and adults, but is seen much less frequently than the norovirus. Sapovirus has been classified into 5 genogroups, but only 4 of them are seen in humans: GI, GII, GIV, and GV.[2]

Adenoviruses are nonenveloped double-stranded DNA viruses. There are approximately 51 different types, but only 3 serotypes (31, 40, and 41) cause gastroenteritis. They typically infect children younger than 2 years and are uncommonly seen in adult shedding, and therefore they are not discussed in this article.

Astrovirus, although seen in children, can also infect adults. Approximately 8 "classic" serotypes are known, with 2 additional types of this single-stranded RNA virus identified recently.[2] Astrovirus infections can occur year-round but like norovirus are most active in the winter months.

Rotavirus is a double-stranded RNA structure subdivided into 7 serogroups, with group A being the most important one for humans. It is seen primarily in children, but adults with close contact with infected children may also become infected.

SYMPTOMS

Norovirus typically starts with nausea and vomiting, followed by abdominal cramping and watery diarrhea. Additional symptoms include fever, chills, fatigue, myalgia, and headaches. Usually the symptoms are self-limiting, with symptomatic early treatment. The incubation period of 1 to 2 days is similar in sapovirus and norovirus, but sapovirus tends to last a little longer (approximately 6 days).

Astroviruses have a short incubation period of 36 to 48 hours, although symptoms may not occur for up to 3 to 4 days after exposure. Diarrhea is the predominant symptom, with some vomiting possible, but symptoms are typically milder than with norovirus or rotavirus. Older adults tend to experience abdominal pain, headache, and nausea with the diarrhea but not vomiting or fever.

Rotavirus has an incubation period of 2 to 6 days, with symptoms lasting 3 to 7 days. The typical diarrhea is associated with abdominal cramps without vomiting. Fever, anorexia, headache, and malaise are common. Generally the symptoms are more severe for children than adults.[1]

Symptoms of dehydration, such as dry mucous membranes, lethargy, hypotension, and oliguria, may not be evident but should be assessed throughout the illness. Gross blood or mucus in the stool is an unusual finding in viral gastroenteritis, and other causes should be considered if present.

TRANSMISSION

Transmission occurs through the fecal-oral route and occurs from person to person, because the virus is present in the stool and vomitus of the infected person, and from contaminated food and water. Infected people can contaminate surfaces, food, drinks, and items in their environment. With vomiting, the virus can become airborne. Therefore, touching contaminated surfaces, sharing of cold food and drink, ingesting contaminated food or water, or even swallowing airborne particles can render a person infected.

A very low infectious dose of only 18 to 20 viral particles makes norovirus gastroenteritis highly contagious from the moment one feels ill until weeks after. The very short incubation period allows for a rapid spread before an outbreak may be considered. Even asymptomatic adults can shed the virus in their stools, thereby unknowingly promoting the spread of infection. The combination of a low infectious dose, viral shedding before and for weeks after illness, and resistance to temperatures from freezing to 60°C and to many common household cleaners makes norovirus a challenge for health care providers.[2] Norovirus can live for months on surfaces until they are disinfected with a bleach solution. Infected people even after symptoms have abated can still spread the infection through their stools for up to 8 weeks.

Since norovirus has been identified, it is clear that it causes most episodes of viral gastroenteritis in adults. In fact, 90% of outbreaks previously of unknown cause are noroviruses.[2] In addition to human costs, economic losses in supplies, closed beds, and staff time off is thought to exceed $650,000 in the United States annually.[4]

New variant strains of norovirus seem to have emerged recently across the world through mutation, much like influenza viruses. These norovirus strains have been associated with an increase in the number of annual outbreaks. In 2002, a genetic shift in circulating strains was noted with the emergence of the GII.4-2002 variant strain.[5] Subsequently, not only was activity higher in the spring but also an unusually high number of outbreaks occurred in the winter season 2002–2003 worldwide.[5] This type of pattern repeated in 2004 with the GII.4-2004 strain and again in 2006 with the GII.4-2006a and GII.4-2006b strains.[5]

Researchers examined the trends in morbidity and mortality based on these gastroenteritis outbreaks in the elderly. Many episodes of gastroenteritis do not result in laboratory testing, so in addition to laboratory surveillance and norovirus outbreak surveillance, they investigated unspecified gastroenteritis in general practitioner office visits and hospital visits, and unspecified gastroenteritis as a primary or secondary cause of death. The trends identified in their research supported their hypothesis that norovirus epidemics are associated with morbidity and mortality in the elderly in Netherlands. These trends may be influenced by the evolution of viruses, and indicate that gastroenteritis should not be taken lightly in the elder population.[5]

Sapovirus is spread similar to norovirus and primarily affects children younger than 5 years. However, it has been found to be spread by asymptomatic adults. It has been spread from infected asymptomatic adult health care workers to elderly patients.[2]

Astrovirus is spread through the fecal-oral route but is uncommon in the adult population, although it has been seen in nosocomial and epidemic diarrhea.[2]

Rotavirus is the most common cause of gastroenteritis in children and affects adults much less frequently. However, approximately one-third of parents of infected children also become infected with rotavirus.[2] Rotavirus outbreaks have occurred in nursing home settings and from contaminated food and water.

Another study examined the causes of gastroenteritis, especially in the elderly, through testing 4024 stool samples collected over 7 seasons. Of these samples, taken from people ages 1 month to 99 years, 1241 were found to contain at least 1 identifiable agent. Rotavirus was the most common causative virus, followed by norovirus.[6] Norovirus, however, was the leading identified virus in all samples from patients aged 6 years and older, with the highest numbers in those older than 65 years.[6] The authors point out that elderly people seem to be more susceptible to norovirus and would benefit from early identification and treatment to avoid outbreaks.

Kirk and colleagues[7] conducted a review of literature describing the epidemiology of gastroenteritis and food-borne illnesses in elderly living in long-term care facilities (LTCFs). Their review showed that enteric infections are primarily acquired from infected persons or contaminated foods, and less often from poor personal hygiene or contaminated environments or water.

DIAGNOSIS

Diagnosis is generally based on symptoms, and in mild cases infected persons may not even contact their health care provider. For severe symptoms lasting several days, health care providers are typically sought out and may test a stool sample to determine the type of virus or to rule out bacterial or parasitic causes. A full diagnostic workup is indicated whenever the following conditions exist: profuse watery diarrhea with signs of hypovolemia (eg, hypotension, tachycardia, pale, clammy, dizziness); small stools with blood or mucus; bloody diarrhea; temperature greater than 38.5°C; passage of greater than 6 unformed stools in 24 hours or illness lasting greater than 48 hours; severe abdominal pain; currently hospitalized or recently taking antibiotics; diarrhea in the elderly or immunocompromised; or systemic illness with diarrhea, especially in pregnant women. Fever may not be present, especially in the elderly. A history of recent food consumption of unpasteurized dairy products, undercooked meat, or seafood is helpful because these are known to be responsible for outbreaks of viral gastroenteritis.

No specific guidelines exist for when to obtain stool cultures. In the elderly, infectious diarrhea may be thought to be fecal incontinence, fecal impaction overflow, irritable bowel syndrome, or even related to a change in medication.[7] In LTCFs, complete surveillance for sporadic disease may be difficult because the patient-to-staff ratio is high and staff may not have the necessary training or experience. If a patient is responding to conservative treatment and avoiding dehydration, samples are usually not obtained. Continuing symptomatic therapy for several days if the patient does not have severe disease is common.

Stool cultures should be obtained on initial presentation for immunocompromised patients, those with significant comorbidities, and those with underlying inflammatory bowel disease. Reverse transcription–polymerase chain reaction (RT-PCR) confirmation is the preferred diagnostic method for these viruses. Stool samples should be collected from infected persons during the acute phase when sensitivity is highest. Some laboratories may require a specific number of suspected cases before sensitivity testing is performed.

A prospective cohort study conducted in Berlin, Germany from August 2005 to August 2007 examined the causes and characteristics of community-acquired acute gastroenteritis in 104 adult patients. In 82% of patients, stool specimens and serologic tests detected enteric pathogens, identified as *Campylobacter* spp (35%), norovirus

(23%), *Salmonella* spp (20%), and rotavirus (15%).[8] The high percentage of severe viral gastroenteritis identified in this study shows the importance of comprehensive microbiologic analysis to support rapid diagnosis and prevention of the spread of infection in hospitalized adults.[8]

Some serologic evidence shows past infection in many young adults, but there is no long-term protective immunity and reinfections are common. Short-term immunity could occur for a few months or up to 1 year, but the immunity is for the specific causative virus and not for any different genotype.

TREATMENT

The goal of treatment is symptom relief and avoiding complications. Most cases do not require specific treatment. Some believe that over-the-counter loperamide and bismuth subsalicylate may help decrease episodes of stooling but should be avoided early in the course to allow for elimination of the virus. Bismuth subsalicylate is believed to reduce the length and severity of abdominal cramping. Antibiotic therapy is not required. Diuretics may need to be omitted for a day or 2 until diarrhea decreases.

Oral rehydration to avoid dehydration should begin as soon as the adult is able to sip clear liquids or suck on ice chips. Once vomiting has ended, fluid intake is encouraged. Reestablishing fluid and electrolyte balance in mild disease can often be accomplished by drinking fruit juices, sports drinks, broths, and caffeine-free soft drinks. High-sugar beverages of any type may increase diarrhea. Small frequent servings of liquids are less likely to increase vomiting than large quantities consumed quickly.

Slow introduction of foods that are bland and easy to digest, such as applesauce, bananas, rice, toast or bread, noodles, and potatoes, helps with symptom relief. Avoiding alcohol, caffeine, and fatty foods until full recovery is advised. Secondary lactose malabsorption is common after infectious gastroenteritis and can last weeks to months. Temporarily avoiding lactose-containing foods may be necessary. Other treatments not routinely used in clinical practice but that have shown some promise in studies to shorten duration or alleviate symptoms include nitazoxanide, antisecretory or toxin-binding agents, and probiotics.[2] More research is needed to determine their usefulness and potential side effects.

COMPLICATIONS

Dehydration is the most common complication experienced by patients with viral gastroenteritis. If the fluid lost through vomiting and diarrhea is not replaced by the patient in the form of oral intake, dehydration will result.

Under normal conditions, the intestine can both absorb and secrete fluids. During a diarrheal illness, a net secretion of fluids occurs because of a failure to absorb fluids normally or because of mucosal injury or toxin-induced excessive secretion.[9] When the colon cannot absorb this excessive fluid, it is excreted as diarrhea. Electrolyte imbalance can result with high-volume diarrhea.

Patients most at risk for dehydration include infants, children, older adults, and anyone with a weakened immune system. Dehydration signs include excessive thirst, dark-colored urine, dry skin and mucous membranes, dizziness or lightheadedness, lethargy, and poor capillary refill. Severe dehydration symptoms include all of these symptoms and weakness, confusion, tachycardia, oliguria, and coma. Severe dehydration is a medical emergency and requires immediate attention. Laboratory abnormalities, such as elevated urine-specific gravity and elevated blood urea nitrogen, may indicate the degree of dehydration. Leukocytosis may be present.

The risk for dehydration is impacted by the severity of the disease, the individual, and the setting in which they are recovering. Elderly persons living alone or in an LTCF often rely on someone else to bring them adequate hydration and monitor them for response. They are clearly a population at risk.

Additionally, dormitory or camp settings where the bathroom and sleeping areas are shared can increase the challenges of confining the disease and those associated with recovery. The embarrassment of frequent vomiting and diarrhea especially when individuals do not feel they have the physical strength to take care of their personal needs adds to the stress of the illness. Recovery from gastroenteritis in this setting in which they are relying on friends to assist them and bring them adequate and appropriate sources of hydration can be problematic. As any of these populations become increasingly weak and tired, they may choose sleep over re-hydration and therefore put themselves at increased risk for dehydration.

Dehydration and hypovolemia are not synonymous. As water is lost from the body's total water, hypernatremia occurs, which is a relative deficit of water in relation to sodium. This condition leads to an intracellular water deficit through the osmotic movement of water into the extracellular fluid, and thus dehydration occurs. Hypovolemia occurs when the extracellular fluid volume is reduced, leading to a shift in intravascular volume, and when severe can cause reduction in tissue perfusion. If significant salt and water loss occurring through diarrhea and vomiting is not replaced, the patient becomes hypovolemic. Thus, patients with severe viral gastroenteritis with a fever, profuse diarrhea, and minimal fluid intake can present with volume depletion evidenced by poor skin turgor, tachycardia, orthostatic changes, and elevated plasma sodium concentration. These patients would have both dehydration and hypovolemia. The intense stimulation of thirst induced by hypernatremia would normally stimulate one to drink, but those with impaired mental status or unable to express their thirst are most at risk.

ORAL REHYDRATION THERAPY FOR MILD TO MODERATE VIRAL GASTROENTERITIS

Oral replacement solutions (ORS) were introduced back in 1945 and were surprisingly similar to some solutions used today. In the 1950s, new commercially prepared solutions were introduced that had too high a carbohydrate level and resulted in multiple episodes of hypernatremia. At that time, ORS were used infrequently and providers relied on intravenous hydration to treat hypovolemia. In the 1960s an effort was undertaken to develop an effective oral rehydration therapy that would be less costly and easy to administer.

In normal adults, the intestine secretes and absorbs a great deal of fluid. Approximately 6500 mL enter the intestine from ingested fluids and secretions combined, and are reduced to approximately 100 mL of stool daily. This passive water absorption is dependent on the osmotic gradient that is dictated by sodium transport via 3 principal mechanisms: sodium/hydrogen exchangers, electrochemical gradient, and sodium-coupled transport with carrier organic solutes such as glucose. In a diarrheal disease such as viral gastroenteritis, many of these processes are disrupted, but the sodium-coupled transport with carrier organic solutes remains intact. This feature is the basis of oral rehydration solutions and how they are effective.

The oral solution used to assist with rehydration must include glucose to allow sodium and water to be transported into the circulation. Without adequate glucose, the solution would not be absorbed and would only contribute to the volume of diarrhea.[9] Likewise, beverages with a higher glucose-to-sodium ratio, such as in fruit juices and soda, will increase diarrheal loss. Therefore, oral rehydration solutions must include glucose and sodium in the correct ratio and be palatable to encourage their consumption. The ORS recommended by the World Health Organization (WHO) and United Nations Children's Fund (UNICEF) for global use is detailed in **Box 1**.

Advantages to ORS include the ability to use it in the home, lower cost, and possible avoidance of a trip to the hospital for intravenous hydration. The WHO-ORS composition is readily available and should be manufactured as a pharmaceutical product. A variety of commercially produced oral rehydration solutions are available over-the-counter.

The electrolyte concentration of sports drinks designed for sweat replacement (such as Gatorade) are not the same as those in oral rehydration solutions. Oral rehydration was the focus of a study by Rao and colleagues[9] examining the efficacy, safety, and palatability of Pedialyte, Gatorade, and a New Oral Rehydration Solution (N-ORS) in an adult population with mild to moderate viral gastroenteritis. This randomized double-blind trial took place in a hospital setting, where they measured stool and urine output, fluid intake, body weight, electrolytes, hematocrit, and palatability. The results showed improved stool frequency, consistency, and body weight in all 3 groups, without differences among groups. All other parameters were similar. Subjects with normal electrolytes on admission were able to maintain them throughout the study, but those with hypokalemia or hyponatremia in the Gatorade group were less likely to correct this imbalance.[9] The authors state that this may be a skewed result because the Gatorade group had a higher percentage of hyponatremic and hypokalemic subjects than the other groups. The subjects preferred the taste of the Gatorade and the N-ORS versus the Pedialyte. The authors discuss the importance of this finding, because a sport drink such as Gatorade tends to be relatively less expensive, available in most convenience stores, and well tolerated by the public. Therefore, Gatorade may be effective in helping to treat dehydration associated with mild viral gastroenteritis. Diluted fruit juices and flavored soda drinks with saltine crackers and broth or soup may help rehydrate those who are less severely ill.

INTRAVENOUS THERAPY FOR SEVERE VIRAL GASTROENTERITIS

It is important to monitor patient progress carefully and consider checking electrolytes when symptoms persist and replace them as appropriate. Intravenous fluids are necessary for those with severe dehydration and hypovolemia.

Box 1
Oral rehydration salts recommended by the WHO and UNICEF for global use

- Total osmolality of 245 mmol/L

- Equimolar concentrations of glucose and sodium

- Glucose, 75 mmol/L

- Sodium, 75 mmol/L

- Potassium, 20 mmol/L

- Citrate, 10 mmol/L

- Chloride, 65 mmol/L

Data from World Health Organization. Oral rehydration salts: production of the new ORS. 2006. Available at: http://whqlibdoc.who.int/hq/2006/WHO_FCH_CAH_06.1.pdf. Accessed March 20, 2012.

Treatment for severe cases of viral gastroenteritis leading to hypovolemia is similar to treating hypovolemia from other causes. Intravenous replacement of fluids should be performed at a rate tolerated by the patient depending on their comorbidities. Those with renal and cardiac dysfunction are more prone to fluid overload and pulmonary edema, and thus monitoring of fluid repletion is critical. They may benefit from a fluid challenge over 1 to 2 hours, and then carefully reassessed through monitoring urine output, blood pressure, heart rate, and mental status. In patients with severe hypovolemia and organ dysfunction, rapid fluid replacement at 200 to 300 mL/h for short periods with frequent reassessments is recommended. The most critically ill patients who develop severe systemic inflammatory response syndrome may benefit from additional close monitoring of central venous pressure and pulmonary central wedge pressure. Gastrointestinal tract losses can be replaced by 5% dextrose in 0.45% sodium chloride, with the addition of potassium as needed to replete to normal levels.

Untreated hypovolemia can result in hypercalcemia, hypernatremia, and azotemia. If allowed to progress, renal failure and cardiac dysrhythmias can occur. Decreased tissue perfusion can lead to worsening of existing comorbid conditions and organ failure.

OUTBREAKS

Viral gastroenteritis outbreaks occur in settings where many people gather together, such as homes, dormitories, cruise ships, restaurants, schools, camps, childcare centers, sporting events, hospitals, military residents, and nursing homes. Many of these patients will end up in emergency departments, and the most vulnerable of them will be admitted.

In 1979–1995, gastroenteritis rates in hospital discharges had decreased in the United States. Lopman and colleagues[10] conducted a study examining gastroenteritis-associated hospital discharges in the United States from 1996–2007. They wanted to determine if the rates had continued to decrease in the setting of increased norovirus activity over recent years. They used the Nationwide Inpatient Sample (NIS) as a nationally representative database of hospital inpatient stays in the United States. They attempted to estimate the proportion of cause-unspecified gastroenteritis codes that were due to norovirus using indirect approaches. They determined that the rate of cause-unspecified gastroenteritis increased by 41% from 1996 to 1997 to 2006 through 2007. Results across age groups revealed a decrease in rates for children but increased by more than 50% for adults and the elderly.[10] Estimates of norovirus-associated hospitalizations and rotavirus-associated activity in nonpediatric age groups increased over the study period.[10] This study highlights the high number of cause-unspecified gastroenteritis and the need for increased diagnostic testing in emergency, inpatient, and LTCF settings. Reliable testing would help to identify and rapidly treat outbreaks.

To determine the importance of norovirus and other enteric viruses as the cause of sporadic and outbreak cases of acute gastroenteritis, Liu et al[4] conducted a study in Beijing, China from July 2007 through June 2008. They examined 557 stool samples consisting of 503 sporadic cases and 54 samples of 4 outbreaks. Their results included detection of norovirus in 26.6% of all cases. Norovirus was present throughout most of the study period but was most evident in the winter and early spring. Norovirus coinfected with rotavirus, astrovirus, and sapovirus. Additionally, the GII.4/2006 genotype was the predominant strain identified.

Outbreaks of norovirus gastroenteritis are especially concerning in vulnerable populations, such as the elderly and individuals who are immunocompromised. Schwartz and colleagues[11] describes an outbreak of norovirus genotype II.4 variant strain in a hematologic and transplantation hospital unit that started from 1 patient with B-cell chronic lymphocytic leukemia who had undergone hematopoietic stem cell transplantation 7 months prior. Stool samples were negative for bacteria and parasites, and the cause of gastrointestinal symptoms was originally thought to be intestinal graft-versus-host disease. Within 6 days of admission, 4 other patients developed vomiting and diarrhea, which prompted laboratory screening for norovirus. In total, 11 patients and 11 staff members contracted norovirus; an attack rate of 3.3% for patients and 10.5% for staff members, which is considered much lower than previously reported rates exceeding 50%. Isolation precautions were followed immediately after norovirus was identified, which may have decreased the attack rate. Staff members were dismissed and did not return to work for 48 hours after symptoms ceased. Stool samples remained positive for norovirus RNA for a median of 30 days, but no transmission was observed after the 48-hour asymptomatic interval.[11] Histo-blood groups and secretor status typing were examined and all 11 infected patients were secretor-positive phenotype; 3 of these patients died.[11] The authors stress the importance of meticulous measures to prevent the transmission of norovirus gastroenteritis to this vulnerable population.

In outbreaks related to contamination of food or water, the source should be identified quickly so that public health measures can be taken immediately. Most foodborne cases of gastroenteritis in the United States are from norovirus and the source is either contaminated food or from infected food handlers themselves.

Outbreaks have even occurred in professional sports organizations. Overall, 21 players and 3 staff members from 13 National Basketball Association (NBA) teams in 11 states were affected by a norovirus outbreak from November to December 2010.[3] Some players identified that a gastrointestinal illness was present in their homes before they became ill. Others described illness occurring in their homes the week after their illness. Both situations indicate the continued spread of this outbreak in otherwise healthy individuals.

A new study approached the topic of frequency of outbreaks by surveying members of the Association for Professionals in Infection Control and Epidemiology about outbreak investigations conducted over the past 24 months in U.S. hospitals. Four organisms were responsible for nearly 60% of all outbreaks reported:

Norovirus (18%)
Staphylococcus aureus (17%)
Acinetobacter spp (14%)
Clostridium difficile (10%)[12]

Norovirus outbreaks occurred more often in rehabilitation, long-term care acute units/hospitals, and behavioral health settings than in medical surgical units, and were associated with the highest number of closures in all settings.[12] The authors concluded that norovirus is emerging as an increasingly common hospital-associated infection that could lead to unit closures.

GENERAL INFECTION PREVENTION MEASURES

In all settings, hand hygiene and disinfecting with bleach solution are important measures to prevent the spread of viral gastroenteritis. After an episode of vomiting or diarrhea, contaminated surfaces should be cleaned and disinfected immediately using a bleach-based household cleaner or an Environmental Protection Agency–approved disinfectant.

Clothing or linens that may be contaminated with vomit or fecal matter must be removed and washed using the maximum cycle length and dried in a machine when possible. Soiled items should be handled carefully to avoid spreading the virus.

Individuals infected with norovirus should not prepare food for others while they have symptoms and for 3 days after they recover from their illness.

INFECTION PREVENTION MEASURES IN HEALTH CARE SETTINGS

The CDC developed recommendations for outbreaks in health care settings to help guide practice. Contact precautions should be initiated immediately and continued for a minimum of 48 hours after symptoms have resolved. These measures should include a single room with a dedicated bathroom. Cohorting patients in multioccupancy rooms or in a designated area may be an alternate strategy when private rooms are not available. Extending the isolation and cohorting is recommended for complex medical patients, such as cardiovascular, renal, autoimmune, and immunocompromised patients, because they may experience prolonged viral shedding.[13] Gloves and gowns should be worn when entering patient rooms. Masks and eye protection are advised when providing direct patient care because of the risk of splashes. Staff who may have had norovirus and have since recovered may be the most appropriate personnel to care for symptomatic patients.

Hand hygiene should be actively promoted for patients, visitors, and health care personnel. Soap and water is recommended after care of infected patients or those suspected and not yet confirmed. Alcohol-based hand sanitizers may be used for other routine hand hygiene but are not believed to be as effective against norovirus.

Food handlers must follow strict hand hygiene practices before any food preparation. Shared food should be removed for patients and staff for the duration of the outbreak. Food handlers who become symptomatic with gastroenteritis should be excused from duty immediately and should not return until asymptomatic for a minimum of 48 hours.

Once an outbreak is recognized, rapid identification and confirmation of suspected persons and notification of an infection preventionist should occur. Organizations should develop policies that will enable them to rapidly make clinical and virologic confirmation of suspected cases. If clinical laboratory testing is not immediately available, Kaplan's clinical and epidemiologic criteria should be used to identify a norovirus gastroenteritis outbreak (**Box 2**). Tracking information about outbreaks should include individuals' name, symptoms, dates of outbreak and resolution, and any diagnostic testing results.

Two or more cases should trigger communication to key stakeholders, including clinical staff, environmental services, laboratory administration, and facility administrators. Outbreaks should be reported to local and state health departments, who will report it to the National Outbreak Reporting System (NORS) and CDC. Timely

---

Box 2
Kaplan's clinical and epidemiologic criteria to identify a norovirus outbreak

1. Vomiting in more than half of symptomatic cases

2. Mean (or median) incubation period of 24 to 48 hours

3. Mean (or median) duration of illness of 12 to 60 hours

4. No bacterial pathogen isolated from stool culture

If all 4 criteria are present, norovirus is highly likely the cause. However, approximately 30% of norovirus outbreaks do not meet these criteria.

From the Centers for Disease Control and Prevention. Key Infection Control Recommendations for the Control of Norovirus Outbreaks in Healthcare Settings. Available at: http://www.cdc.gov/HAI/organisms/norovirus.html. Accessed January 16, 2012.

communication to staff and visitors is essential to decrease panic and to further prevent the spread of the virus.

The CDC encourages organizations to use the NORS (http://www.cdc.gov/outbreaknet/nors/) for reporting incidence and fluctuations in norovirus in health care settings.[13] This surveillance program was previously used for reporting foodborne disease only but has been expanded to include any enteric outbreak. In addition, the CDC started CaliciNet, a national surveillance system for genetic sequences of noroviruses that may be used to track changes in the epidemiology of health care–associated norovirus infections.[13]

All organizations should have sick leave policies and they should be followed at this time. Staff should not return until they are asymptomatic for 48 hours. Students, volunteers, and any staff not needed for day-to-day management of patient care should be encouraged to avoid the setting until the outbreak has passed. Group activities are generally canceled during outbreaks, and movement in and out of the patient care area should be discouraged.

Education of staff, patients, and visitors is essential and should include recognition of norovirus symptoms, modes of transmission, prevention of infection, and special considerations for outbreaks. Having resources available for visitors to read in clear simple language will help disseminate the information. Allowing all staff and visitors to have access to personal protective equipment supports the process.

Many organizations have open visitation policies, but should include information regarding limiting visitors during episodes of outbreak. The team will need to screen visitors to determine if they are asymptomatic and encourage them to follow strict hand hygiene practices and contact precautions.

The frequency of cleaning should be increased, and high-touch areas, including door handles, faucets, commodes, toilets, hand/bed railing, telephones, computer equipment, and kitchen preparation areas, require special attention with approved cleaning products. The regular cleaning of the environment should be increased to twice a day, and 3 times a day for high-touch surfaces.[13] The process of cleaning should always be from low contaminated areas such as table tops to high contaminated areas such as commodes and faucets.

Equipment that is shared among patients should always be cleaned with Environmental Protection Agency–registered products, paying special attention to the directions for application and contact time, defined as the time the product must be left on the soiled surface.

When a patient is ready for discharge or transfer, the room should undergo a final cleaning, with all disposable items discarded. Unused linens should be removed and laundered. Nurses can minimize waste through limiting the number of items to those needed and not storing extras in the room.

Cleaning up after an outbreak forces the team to take a look at the environment. All furniture should be able to withstand routine cleaning and disinfecting. Privacy curtains should be removed and laundered. If upholstered furniture is in the patient care area, it should be spot cleaned with an approved product when soiled and then steam cleaned when the patient is transferred or discharged. More research is needed to determine how effective and reliable fogging, ultraviolet irradiation, and ozone mists are in reducing norovirus environmental contamination.[13]

FUTURE RESEARCH

Much still must be learned about these viruses, and specifically about the best strategies to use for controlling the spread of infection. Improvement in detecting causes of gastroenteritis during outbreaks is imperative, because nearly 25% have an unidentified cause using the most sensitive methods available. Braham and colleagues[14] examined a panel of samples from outbreaks of gastroenteritis that had no identified cause and applied random amplification molecular methods. Virus purification and concentration followed by a single-primer sequence-independent amplification method identified viruses in 5 of 51 previously negative outbreaks. Noroviruses were detected in 4 of these outbreaks that were not identified using 2 available broadly reactive diagnostic methods.[14] This study highlights the potential for future methods of early detection.

Protective immunity and the development of a vaccine for norovirus are current areas of focus for researchers. It is known that histo-blood group antigens (HBGAs) help determine host susceptibility for norovirus infection, and individuals with blood type B or AB are less susceptible to norovirus infections. Additionally, Northern Europeans and Americans from Northern European ancestors lack the fucosyl-transferase 2 enzyme and do not express the H type 1 or Lewis b antigens on their mucosae or in secretions.[15] Reeck and colleagues[15] developed an HBGA blocking assay and wanted to examine the ability of human serum to block interaction of norovirus virus–like particles with H type 1 and 3 glycans. Volunteers were inoculated with norovirus and evaluated. Infected individuals had a peak in blocking titers at 28 days after challenge, and these were higher than in those who developed gastroenteritis.[15] They concluded that blocking antibodies correlate with protection against clinical norovirus gastroenteritis.[15] This information can be used in the development of new vaccines.

Other important research topics are length of shedding of virus after symptoms subside and the likelihood of secondary transmission of norovirus infection; the use of medications that may decrease severity and length of disease; the most important risk factors to consider; and treatment options for severe cases of viral gastroenteritis. All of these factors would have significant impact on the control of this and potentially other viruses.

SUMMARY

Viral gastroenteritis is extremely common, causing millions of cases of diarrhea in all age groups worldwide. Norovirus has been identified as the leading cause of viral gastroenteritis in the adult population. The combination of a low infectious dose, viral shedding before and for weeks after illness, and resistance to temperatures from freezing to 60°C and to many common household cleaners makes norovirus a winter peril. Mild cases require symptomatic treatment alone. Complicated cases, often involving the most vulnerable populations, develop severe dehydration and hypovolemia, requiring the skills of critical care nurses to meet the challenges of care.

REFERENCES

1. Viral gastroenteritis. National Digestive Diseases Information Clearinghouse Web site. Available at: http://digestive.niddk.nih.gov/ddiseases/pubs/viralgastroenteritis/. Accessed February 20, 2012.
2. Eckardt AJ, Baumgart DC. Viral gastroenteritis in adults. Recent Pat Antiinfect Drug Discov 2011;6(1):54–63.
3. Viral gastroenteritis. Centers for Disease Control and Prevention Web site. Available at: http://www.cdc.gov/ncidod/dvrd/revb/gastro/faq.htm. Accessed February 20, 2012.
4. Liu LJ, Liu W, Liu YX, et al. Identification of norovirus as the top enteric viruses detected in adult cases with acute gastroenteritis. Am J Trop Med Hyg 2010; 82(4):717–22.

5. van Asten L, Siebenga J, van den Wijngaard C, et al. Unspecified gastroenteritis illness and deaths in the elderly associated with norovirus epidemics. Epidemiology 2011;22(3):336–43.
6. Fernandez J, de Ona M, Melon S, et al. Noroviruses as cause of gastroenteritis in elderly patients. Aging Clin Exp Res 2011;23(2):145–7.
7. Kirk MD, Veitch MG, Hall GV. Gastroenteritis and food-borne disease in elderly people living in long-term care. Clin Infect Dis 2010;50(3):397–404.
8. Jansen A, Stark K, Kunkel J, et al. Aetiology of community-acquired, acute gastroenteritis in hospitalised adults: a prospective cohort study. BMC Infect Dis 2008;8:143.
9. Rao SS, Summers RW, Rao GR, et al. Oral rehydration for viral gastroenteritis in adults: a randomized, controlled trial of 3 solutions. JPEN J Parenter Enteral Nutr 2006;30(5):433–9.
10. Lopman BA, Hall AJ, Curns AT, et al. Increasing rates of gastroenteritis hospital discharges in US adults and the contribution of norovirus, 1996-2007. Clin Infect Dis 2011;52(4):466–74.
11. Schwartz S, Vergoulidou M, Schreier E, et al. Norovirus gastroenteritis causes severe and lethal complications after chemotherapy and hematopoietic stem cell transplantation. Blood 2011;117(22):5850–6.
12. Rhinehart E, Walker S, Murphy D, et al. Frequency of outbreak investigations in US hospitals: results of a national survey of infection preventionists. Am J Infect Control 2012;40(1):2–8.
13. MacCannell T, Umscheid CA, Agarwal RK, et al. Guidelines for the prevention and control of norovirus gastroenteritis outbreaks in healthcare settings. Infect Control Hosp Epidemiol 2012.
14. Braham S, Iturriza-Gomara M, Gray J. Optimisation of a single-primer sequence-independent amplification (SP-SIA) assay: detection of previously undetectable norovirus strains associated with outbreaks of gastroenteritis. J Virol Methods 2009;158(1–2):30–4.
15. Reeck A, Kavanagh O, Estes MK, et al. Serological correlate of protection against norovirus-induced gastroenteritis. J Infect Dis 2010;202(8):1212–8.

Respiratory Syncytial Virus Bronchiolitis in Children

Judy Trivits Verger, RN, PhD, CRNP[a,b,c,*],
Emily Elizabeth Verger, RN, BSN[d]

KEYWORDS

- Bronchiolitis • Respiratory syncytial virus • Respiratory infection

KEY POINTS

- Respiratory syncytial virus is a highly infectious virus that causes high morbidity and a low, but important, incidence of mortality.
- Hydration, nutrition and respiratory support, and airway clearance are supportive measures. Chest physiotherapy, bronchodilators, steroids, and antibiotics have not been associated with significantly improved outcomes.
- Vaccination is the single most effective approach to controlling the spread of disease.

BACKGROUND

Bronchiolitis is an infection in the small airways that leads to obstruction of the lower respiratory tract. The main source of bronchiolitis in humans, and the most common cause of hospitalization in infants and young children, is respiratory syncytial virus (RSV).[1,2] Close to 70% of young infants are infected during their first winter.[3,4] Maternal antibodies fluctuate seasonally and provide partial protection for the very young from significant disease.[5] By the second year of life, 90% of children may be infected at least once, resulting in a large burden of disease worldwide.[1,4,6] Of those children exposed to RSV for the first time 25% to 40% show signs of pneumonia or bronchiolitis.[4,7] Approximately 3% to 10% of children with RSV are hospitalized, depending on age and the patient's comorbidities.[8,9] In Europe, up to 40% of admissions for acute respiratory infection in children less than 2 years of age are attributed to

The authors have nothing to disclose.
[a] Pediatric Critical Care and Neonatal Nurse Practitioner Programs, School of Nursing, Fagin Hall, 418 Curie Boulevard, University of Pennsylvania, Philadelphia, PA 19104, USA; [b] Neonatal and Pediatric Clinical Nurse Specialist Programs, School of Nursing, Fagin Hall, 418 Curie Boulevard, University of Pennsylvania, Philadelphia, PA 19104, USA; [c] Critical Care – Sedation/Radiology, Children's Hospital of Philadelphia, 34th and Civic Center Boulevard, Philadelphia, PA 19104, USA; [d] Neurology and General Pediatrics, Children's Hospital of Philadelphia, 34th and Civic Center Boulevard, Philadelphia, PA 19104, USA
* Corresponding author. Children's Hospital of Philadelphia, 34th and Civic Center Boulevard, Philadelphia, PA 19104, USA.
E-mail address: jtv@nursing.upenn.edu

Crit Care Nurs Clin N Am 24 (2012) 555–572
http://dx.doi.org/10.1016/j.ccell.2012.07.008
0899-5885/12/$ – see front matter © 2012 Elsevier Inc. All rights reserved.

RSV.[10] Critical care services are required for 1% of children with RSV, with a mean length of stay of 2 to 10 days and a median duration of mechanical ventilation of 4.4 days.[11,12] RSV causes as many as 200 to 500 inpatient and outpatient deaths each year.[2,12,13] RSV is estimated to cost health care providers $500 million to $700 million dollars annually.[14,15] For parents of patients admitted to the intensive care unit (ICU), 32% missed work for an average of 3 days.[11]

SCIENCE OF RSV

RSV gets its name from the impact of the virus on respiratory function and the cytopathology of the virus in cell culture, which includes multinucleated cells or syncytia.[3] RSV is a single-stranded negative-polarity protein virus that is a member of the Paramyxoviridae family.[4,13] The virus is an enveloped RNA virus with a single serotype and 2 antigenic subgroups, A and B. RSV interacts with the plasma membrane via viral cell fusion and replication. The genome for RSV was sequenced in 1997 and includes 10 viral genes encoding 11 proteins including RSV proteins involved in nucleocapsid structure and/or RNA synthesis and proteins associated with the lipid bilayer that forms the viral envelop.[4,16] Two glycoproteins, F and G, on the cell surface are known to facilitate replication of the virus. The G glycoprotein is the major attachment protein to connect to the cytoplasm where replication occurs. The fusion protein F directs and penetrates the cell. Neighboring cells are infected through formation of syncytia. The life of the virus begins with attachment of the G protein to the cell membrane followed by F protein–mediated fusion.

As a pathogen, RSV affects airway epithelium and is a driver for airway inflammation, acute lung injury, and the accumulation and activation of lung natural killer cells.[4,17] Infection is typically restricted to the superficial epithelial cells in the respiratory tract. Cell-to-cell transfer occur as the virus moves from the nasal mucosa down the respiratory tract. Ciliated cells of the small bronchioles and type 1 pneumocytes in the alveoli are targeted in the lower respiratory tract.[4] Early inflammatory mediators such as tumor necrosis factor α (TNFa), eotaxin, and interleukin 8 are involved in disease progression.[18,19] RSV infection brings a cellular and humoral immune response.[16,18] Activated T cells are recruited into the lung and promote inflammation. Increased mucus production and sloughing of fibrous and epithelial cells occur. Mucus plugs cause air trapping and obstruction in the bronchioles.

TRANSMISSION

As an airborne disease, RSV is transmitted through droplets and particles by direct and indirect contact.[7,20] A mist of noxious particles is created when people with RSV cough, sneeze, or breathe.[7] Transmission is primarily through direct contact with infected respiratory secretions. RSV can also land on surfaces such as hands and be transmitted to another host. Indirect transmission may occur by fomites, inanimate objects that transmit disease, such as bedside tables and doorknobs. RSV is stable in the environment and the virus can survive on hard surfaces for up to 6 hours.[7]

The start of RSV season is defined by the Centers for Disease Control and Prevention (CDC) as the time in which positive antigen tests are greater than 10% of those sampled.[7] The reasons for outbreak variations are unclear but likely associated with conditions that affect virus viability, population immunity, and circumstances that promote transmission such as population density.[21] In the United States, annual outbreaks occur in fall, winter, and early spring and typically last 5 to 6 months, with some variation by region and year.[7] Florida is an exception, with RSV detected all year, with earlier epidemic onset and peak, and a season that lasts longer than other states .[22] In tropical climates, the occurrence of RSV is less temporally focused, but the incidence is greatest throughout the rainy season.[1] Outbreaks from both RSV strains A and B occur concurrently. However, group A is typically predominant in most seasons and is associated with a greater disease severity.[23] Current surveillance data are available on the CDC Web site and updated biweekly.[24]

RSV is a highly infectious disease in any setting. Children who are otherwise healthy are contagious for approximately 2 to 8 days, whereas those with compromised immune systems may be contagious for as many as 3 weeks.[16] Approximately 50% to 60% of parents and siblings show symptoms of RSV at the same time as their infected child.[7,11] Although associated with a decrease in severity, RSV can reinfect the child during the same hospitalization, in the same season, and from year to year.[4,16] In the ICU, developing nosocomial RSV infections is a major concern.[25,26] Those children with nosocomial RSV have a longer length of stay than those patients with the community-acquired virus.[26]

RISK FACTORS

Chronic and congenital conditions add to the risk of disease severity for children with RSV.[27] Children with congenital heart disease (CHD) and congestive heart failure, pulmonary hypertension, or cyanosis are 2 to 5 times more likely to need critical care services, 30% more likely to be supported with mechanical ventilation, and have double the lengths of hospital stay as children without risk factors.[27-29] Infants with immature lung development and children with lung disease have an increased need for mechanical ventilation, prolonged lengths of stay, and increased admission to the ICU.[27,28,30] Infants born early also have an added likelihood of RSV-related hospitalization, longer lengths of stay, and more admissions to critical care areas independent of lung disease.[11,27,28] In a study of premature infants, more than 8% of subjects with RSV died.[31] A recent investigation found that children with Down syndrome have a higher risk of symptoms and are more frequently hospitalized.[32] Immunocompromised patients also have longer lengths of stay and an increased risk of death compared with nonimmunocompromised patients.[33] Children with neuromuscular disorders who are hospitalized with RSV are more likely to require mechanical ventilation and ICU admission than children without such impairments.[34] In addition, children with a comorbidity are more likely to acquire nosocomial infections.[25,26] Thornburn and colleagues[26] (2004) reported that 73% of children in their ICU had CHD, chronic lung disease, airway abnormalities, or immunosuppression. For those patients with CHD and acquired RSV, 96% were ventilated with 2 requiring extracorporeal membrane oxygenation (ECMO).[26]

Despite the added risk associated with congenital and chronic conditions, two-thirds of children hospitalized with RSV are previously healthy.[12] Certain environmental conditions, patient and family attributes, and genetic predispositions seem to add risk for illness severity without underlying disease. Living with preschool and school-aged siblings and sleeping in a bedroom with 2 or more people may contribute to RSV severity, whereas overall household crowding as an independent variable does not seem to increase RSV risk.[12,25,35,36] Exposure to smoke or other factors that result in poor air quality have resulted in an increased risk for RSV in some studies but not others.[12] RSV was not consistently associated with day care attendance except in a Canadian study that found significant risk for hospitalization of children of 33 to 35 weeks' gestation.[12,36-38]

Age, gender, weight, nutrition, and ethnicity seem to affect RSV incidence and severity. Infants who are young and are less than 6 to 12 months of age at the beginning of viral season have a higher incidence of RSV.[39,40] Boys are more susceptible than girls to RSV.[11] El Saleeby and colleagues[41] (2011) also concluded that a lower admission weight for infants with RSV is a predictor of admission, duration of hospitalization, and respiratory failure. Lack of breastfeeding has also been identified as an independent predictor of hospitalization and more severe disease.[12,41] Belderbos and colleagues[42] (2011) found that neonates with vitamin D deficiency had a 6-fold increased risk for RSV, leading some to think that supplementing vitamin D during pregnancy may reduce RSV infections. Certain groups in various geographic regions also seem to have a higher incidence of RSV with more severe symptoms. American Indian and Alaska Natives with RSV have a higher illness severity than other populations.[43] Some reports have also identified African American ethnicity as a risk factor.[41,44] In addition, genetic features may play a part in the clinical presentation and outcomes of certain infectious diseases like RSV. Native response genes have been associated with susceptibility to RSV, suggesting that approximately 15% of disease severity may be decided by the child's genetics.[45] Viral load and delayed viral clearance seem to affect clinical course. Increased viral load and delayed viral clearance are associated with hospitalization.[41] Greater disease severity, admission to a critical care area, and duration of hospitalization are linked to viral load.[23,41]

CLINICAL PRESENTATION

Children with RSV bronchiolitis often start with coldlike symptoms including rhinorrhea, cough, sneezing, fever, and lethargy. Rhinorrhea usually develops in 2 to 6 days after exposure, with coughing and sneezing to follow about 1 to 3 days later.[7,16] Symptoms typically last 1 to 2 weeks.[7] Fever is reported in 69% of patients with RSV.[12] These symptoms may lead to lethargy and interfere with the child's ability and willingness to eat and drink. As the disease progresses, children can exhibit increasing tachypnea, nasal flaring, and intercostal, subcostal, and substernal retractions.[46] Because infants are obligate nose breathers, mucus in the upper airway may cause significant distress. Apnea is a common complication in infants with RSV and may result in death.[25,47] Bronchospasm may also occur, causing hyperinflation of the lungs, atelectasis, and diffuse wheezing. Levin and colleagues[48] (2008) reported that patients admitted to the ICU have wheezing, grunting, retractions, increased respiratory rate, abnormal blood gases, and variations in their chest radiographs. Long term, an association between RSV and recurrent wheezing and reactive airway disease has been reported after RSV infection.[49] The cause of this association is unclear and may be causative or attributed to the predisposition to exacerbations.[4,49–51]

DIAGNOSIS AND DETECTION

Making the diagnosis of either viral or bacterial infection is paramount to initiating appropriate therapies. The differential diagnosis of viral bronchiolitis includes pneumonia, asthma, foreign body aspiration, pulmonary aspiration, and airway malacia, including bronchomalacia. A comprehensive history and physical examination is the foundation of verifying RSV bronchiolitis. The American Academy of Pediatrics (AAP) suggests that diagnosis for most patients can be based exclusively on the history and physical examination.[52] A history of preexisting conditions that increase risk for disease severity, such as immunodeficiency and prematurity, should be noted. Information regarding the duration and progression of symptoms, feeding behavior, number of wet diapers, and infectious contacts are also solicited. On physical examination, tachypnea, fever, and use of accessory muscles are important findings. On auscultation, crackles with recurrent wheezing may be the predominant feature of bronchiolitis. Increased work of breathing and decreased oral intake leading to dehydration often requires hospitalization.

For children with progressive respiratory failure, a chest radiograph may be indicated. When bronchioles become completely obstructed, air trapping can occur, resulting in patchy atelectasis or infiltrates.[53] It may be difficult to differentiate atelectasis from focal infiltrates attributed to pneumonia. Hyperinflation secondary to increased airway resistance and peribronchial thickening may also be seen.[16,54] When diagnosis is questionable or there is a suspicion of bacterial infection, a complete blood count with differential may be of benefit.

Several techniques in specimen analysis are available to confirm the diagnosis of RSV infection.[55] The sensitivity and specificity of the technique to detect viral load depend on specimen source, collection technique, and patient characteristics.[3,56] Specimen sampling occurs via nasal wash, nasal swab, or airway aspirate.[6,41,57] Although cell culture is the gold standard, rapid diagnosis has benefits including the timely initiation of infection control measures.[7] A reduction in hospital stay and antibiotic use has been noted with rapid diagnostic techniques as evaluated against viral culture.[58] The reported sensitivity of antigen assays generally ranges from 80% to 90% compared with cell culture.[7,59] Direct fluorescent antibody (DFA) detection provides more rapid results but is less sensitive than viral culture.[60] Polymerase chain reaction (PCR) assays are also available for exposing respiratory pathogens and are often more sensitive than tissue culture and antigen detections tests.[55] PCR may be the best alternative for older children because of the low viral loads typically seen in older children and adults.[55,61] Results can be obtained within 6 to 24 hours but lead to increased expense without reduction in antibiotic use compared with DFA.[41,62,63] Although useful for seroprevalence and epidemiologic studies, antibody titers via serology testing are less helpful for individual patients and therefore less frequently used for routine diagnosis. The delay in receiving results for serology testing makes it less likely to guide patient care in a timely manner.

PREVENTION

Preventing the spread of RSV is critically important and should be a priority concern. Prevention depends on infection control and purposeful approaches to hygiene, as well as prophylaxis for vulnerable infants.[64] Hand hygiene with alcohol-based hand sanitizer or antimicrobial soap and water before and after contact with the child is vital. Hands are a vehicle for RSV transmission, making hand washing essential for every caregiver. Contact isolation is part of the mainstay of infection control procedures, with gowns and gloves desirable when in close contact with the patient.[53] During hospitalization, patients with RSV may be cohorted and visitors screened to prevent the spread of RSV.[64] During times when RSV is widespread, limiting contact with visitors is appropriate. Staff education is also an essential component of containing RSV infection. In response to an increased incidence of hospital-acquired RSV, reinforcement of basic droplet safety measures was reported by 1 pediatric ICU (PICU) as the solution to a breakdown in barrier precautions.[26]

Palivizumab (Synagis) is a neutralizing humanized monoclonal antibody that binds and envelops the fusion glycoprotein of RSV.[65] Since 1998, palivizumab has been approved to establish passive immunity against RSV-specific antibodies, replacing RSV-IGIV (Respigram).[66] Palivizumab is currently recommended for children at high risk for severe illness to reduce severity of illness and hospitalization.[7] Eligible children are determined by gestational age, age at the beginning of RSV season, pertinent diagnosis, and presence of risk factors.[7] The IMpact-RSV study established that monthly intramuscular injections could reduce hospitalization for children with chronic lung disease and prematurity.[66] In addition, children with CHD and hemodynamic instability, including congestive heart failure, pulmonary hypertension, and cyanosis, have a 45% decrease in RSV-related hospitalization.[67] In response to additional evidence, the AAP recommendations for palivizumab were expanded in 2003 and 2009 to include patients with conditions that compromise immune function and for infants during the first year of life who have airway and congenital neuromuscular anomalies.[7]

Palivizumab prophylaxis is optimally started before exposure to RSV and administered monthly (every 28–30 days) with a maximum of 3 to 5 doses depending on condition.[64] The AAP recommends a start date of November 1 in all states except Florida.[52] The administration of palivizumab during hospitalization has also shown a reduction in nosocomial infections. When used in neonatal ICUs, outbreaks of RSV can be controlled.[68–70] In addition, palivizumab has been reported to reduce subsequent recurrent wheezing in premature infants.[71] Motazvizumab, a high-affinity derivative of palivizumab, also produced positive immunoprophylaxis in otherwise healthy and high-risk infants.[72–74] However, motavizumab production was suspended in 2010 because it offers no advantage compared with palivizumab.[75]

Despite its clinical effectiveness, several factors affect routine palivizumab administration.[76,77] The cost of palivizumab is high and its cost-effectiveness has been questioned.[68,75,76] Given the expensive nature of the drug, its unlimited use is not indicated. In addition, several have reported confusion regarding the AAP guidelines for identifying eligible patients and fulfilling recommendations.[31,77,78] Additional ongoing challenges are the use of palivizumab outside the guidelines and inadequate dosing. Sampalis[31] (2003) reported that fewer than 50% of those eligible for palivizumab are receiving appropriate immunoprophylaxis. In addition, Perrin and Begue[77] (2012) found that only 29% of eligible children received the appropriate number of doses. Compliance is especially low in Medicaid patients and patients of minority decent.[79] In addition, parental perception of benefit, language difficulties, and limited access based on inadequate transportation and other issues affected compliance. Continued education of providers is warranted.

Vaccination is the single most effective approach to controlling spread of infectious disease.[16] Past and current efforts have produced a plethora of candidates to provide protection from RSV.[13] Despite this, a vaccine for RSV has not yet been developed that provides adequate antibody titers. Scientific confounders, as well as overcoming the challenges of testing a vaccine in a vulnerable infant population, contribute to the lack of success. New approaches to vaccine development continue to be pursued, with one author speculating that a vaccine may be available within 5 to 10 years.[13]

MANAGEMENT

Whether at home or hospitalized, supportive care is the basis of treatment.[80] Respiratory support and hydration/nutrition management are the primary therapeutic strategies for children with bronchiolitis.[81] For many children, RSV is self-limiting and can be adequately treated at home. However, hospitalization and ICU admission are required for a noteworthy number of young children with the most severe disease.[1,6,12,82]

Respiratory assessment and support are the cornerstones of RSV management. Hall and coleagues[12] (2009) found that 95% of patients hospitalized with RSV had labored respirations and required oxygen. Ongoing assessment to establish a need for escalation in services is essential. Cardiopulmonary monitoring is especially important for those children at risk for apnea and impending respiratory failure.[80] Pulse oximetry may be a helpful adjunct in detecting hypoxemia suspected on physical examination. For infants with a natural airway, nasal suctioning is often indicated to ensure that the nasal passage is clear.[83] For the child with decreasing oxygen saturation (SpO_2), using supplemental oxygen to maintain an SpO_2 of more than 92% to 95% is recommended.[52]

For those children who cannot maintain adequate oxygenation, noninvasive positive pressure ventilation (NIPPV) may be necessary.[84] Nasal continuous positive airway pressure (CPAP) is widely accepted as an effective ventilatory support method before or after mechanical ventilation in severe bronchiolitis by keeping the airway open and improving alveolar ventilation and clinical outcome.[85–87] By recruiting collapsed alveoli and related airways, complete exhalation is achieved and hyperinflation and work of breathing decreases.[88,89] Essouri and colleagues[90] (2011) found that nasal CPAP is associated with an immediate improvement in breathing pattern and respiratory muscle pattern. Nasal CPAP supports infants because they are obligate nose breathers. The optimal level of CPAP is reported as 7 cm H_2O to support breathing in severe bronchiolitis.[90] Despite its effect on gas exchange and work of breathing, there is no conclusive evidence that CPAP reduces the need for intubation.[88] However, higher levels of CPAP may increase gastric pressure from air spillage into the stomach and may have a deleterious effect on the work of breathing.[90] Given that infants are obligate nose breathers, a high-flow nasal cannula or CPAP may be especially helpful in this age group.

Heliox, an inert gas composed of helium and oxygen, is a popular therapeutic adjunct in the care of severe bronchiolitis. As a low-density gas, heliox decreases the resistance of gas flow and reduces the work of breathing.[89,91] In a meta-analysis of patients with bronchiolitis admitted to the PICU, Liet and colleagues[92] (2010) found that heliox improved respiratory status after 1 hour of therapy. Despite an association between heliox and improved $PaCO_2$ and work of breathing, there is no substantive evidence that heliox alone reduces the need for intubation.[85,88,92–94]

For those children with continuing deterioration and impending respiratory failure, positive pressure mechanical ventilation may be required.[27,95] A tidal volume (TV) of 6 to 8 mL/kg with a peak end expiratory pressure (PEEP) of 3 to 4 cm H_2O has been used as a guide to support adequate ventilation in children with RSV bronchiolitis.[48] Maintaining a peak inspiratory pressure (PIP) of less than 20 to 30 cm H_2O may also help over-distention in infants with poor compliance.[96] For those children who need additional lung protection, a smaller TV and PIP can be combined with higher PEEP.[95] The age-appropriate respiratory rate can guide the set mechanical breathing rate with modifications made to meet individual patient needs. Other modalities of ventilation, such as high frequency jet ventilation and high-frequency oscillatory ventilation, may be used to promote gas exchange. These high-frequency ventilatory modes support oxygenation by recruiting lung volume with high mean airway pressures and low TV and changes in airway pressure.[96] ECMO, inhaled nitric oxide, and the administration of natural surfactant has also been used with some success in children with bronchiolitis.[48,97]

The usefulness of hypertonic saline with and without other aerosolized medications has been evaluated for the treatment of bronchiolitis.[80,98,99] Nebulized 3% normal saline administered with bronchodilators decreased length of stay by 26% in some patients.[100] Suggested mechanisms of action for hypertonic saline include facilitating drainage by softening secretions, stimulating cough, and reducing edema in the submucosal tissue by absorbing water from the mucosa and supporting the functioning of airway cilia.[99]

Ribavirin, an antiviral medication, is the only treatment approved by the US Food and Drug Administration for targeted treatment of RSV. Ribavirin is a synthetic nucleoside with broad antiviral activity that interferes with the RNA metabolism required for replication of viral genetic material. Typically, ribavirin is administered aerosolized for approximately 12 or more hours a day for 3 to 7 days.[54] Hemolytic anemia is the most common side effect and is particularly problematic for patients with cardiac conditions. For health care workers, there is concern for the toxic effects of ribavirin related to exposure to the aerosolized medication. Despite the conclusion of a 2007 Cochrane Report that ribavirin may reduce the duration of mechanical ventilation and days of hospitalization, its efficacy in children has been questioned.[101] In 2010, Ventre and Randolph,[102] the investigators of the original analysis, withdrew the report, indicating that ribavirin trials "lack sufficient power to provide reliable estimates of its effect."[102] In patients following lung transplant, oral and intravenous (IV) ribavirin have been well tolerated and effective.[103,104] Given that ribavirin is expensive with modest effects, its use is limited.[80] The AAP suggests that priority administration be given to newborns and infants and children with potentially life-threatening disease.[43]

Ensuring adequate hydration and nutrition is central to the care of children with RSV. For those children with significant work of breathing or dehydration, IV hydration may be necessary. Standard isotonic IV fluids with a dextrose and sodium chloride solution are typically sufficient. For most patients, infusing fluids at a maintenance rate provides adequate hydration. For patients with significant hypovolemia, administering added volume with normal saline or lactated ringers may be necessary. Fever may also contribute to increases in water loss, and treatment with dose-appropriate ibuprofen or acetaminophen is recommended.

Nutrition is very important for infants and children because of their high metabolic demands and limited energy stores. Delayed initiation of feeding and subsequent interruptions contribute to suboptimal nutrition and should be avoided.[105] The metabolic stress of illness and an inadequate supply of nutrients can cause malnutrition.[106] Poor nutrition may contribute to physiologic instability and result in a negative impact on growth.[107] For children with significant respiratory distress, oral feeding may not be possible. Nutritional needs can be met by enteral nutrition (EN) or parenteral nutrition (PN), or a combination of both.[108] In general, EN is well tolerated by critically ill children and is the preferred feeding route.[109] To provide adequate calories, a gastric or postpyloric feeding tube can be placed. Although gastric feeding is more physiologic, postpyloric feeding may be the better alternative because of the reduced gastric residuals and less frequent interruptions. Zamberlan and colleagues[107] (2011) reported that as many as 40% of PICU patients receive postpyloric EN. Although technically more difficult, nasojejunal feeding tubes can be placed successfully at the bedside.[110] Depending on the route (gastric vs postpyloric), continuous or intermittent delivery options are available. Both delivery methods yield the same prevalence of feeding intolerance as defined by vomiting and diarrhea.[111] For infants, breast milk is ideal.[52,80] If breast milk is not possible, offering infants their regular formula is usually adequate. Specialized formulations of EN are also available for pediatric patients. Although IV nutrition comes with a higher risk of infection, PN should be initiated for seriously ill pediatric patients who are unable to receive adequate calories from EN. Standard formulas are available that are configured to meet the unique needs of infants and children.[112]

Therapies with Insufficient Evidence

Conventional chest physiotherapy (CPT) and the use of bronchodilators, steroids, and other medications have not been associated with significantly improved outcomes for children with RSV bronchiolitis.[43,80] CPT with standard percussion, vibration, and cough assist has no effect on duration of illness or duration of hospitalization.[113,114] A 2011 investigation evaluating an alternative CPT method that included prolonged slow expiration and provoked cough found only short-term improvement of wheezing.[115] Given the insufficient evidence, conventional CPT cannot be recommended as a standard of care for patients with uncomplicated RSV.[80]

No substantive evidence supports significant beneficial effects of bronchodilators alone in children with bronchiolitis.[52,80,116] Regardless of the evidence, clinicians continue to use β2 agonists, epinephrine, and anticholinergics for wheezing secondary to bronchiolitis, presumably because of their effectiveness in the treatment of asthma.[117] An evaluation of bronchodilators including epinephrine, levalbuterol, and albuterol was undertaken in 2008 of mechanically ventilated infants.[48] Although there were small short-term improvements in PIP, all groups, including those infants who received inhaled saline, had a meaningful decrease in airway resistance. In addition, those treated with bronchodilators had significant increase in heart rate, making the cost/benefit and efficacy of bronchodilators questionable. In addition, a 2010 Cochrane Review found no improvement in oxygen saturation, no reduction in hospital admission after outpatient treatment, and no decrease in hospitalization length of stay.[116] A systematic review of epinephrine with and without dexamethasone did conclude that some short-term benefits exist for outpatients with bronchiolititis.[118] For a small group of infants, the AAP maintains that a trial of bronchodilators is a reasonable approach to RSV treatment, with continuation based on the clinical improvement of the child.[52]

Montelukast (Singular) therapy has also been shown by some (but not by others) to improve respiratory symptoms including wheezing and coughing.[119,120] In theory, this leukotriene receptor antagonist may have benefit because leukotrienes are found in the airways of infants with RSV bronchiolitis.[54] A recent study published in the *Journal of Pediatrics* found that infants with RSV bronchiolitis after receiving montelukast had lower eosinophil-derived neurotoxin levels with significantly less reoccurring episodes of wheezing after receiving montelukast.[121] However, a large randomized multisite trial of nearly 1000 children less than 24 months old found no difference in symptom-free days when comparing montelukast with placebo. Because of the limited and questionable effects of montelukast it is currently not recommended as a standard of care.[80]

The use of steroids in the treatment of bronchiolitis has also been investigated.[122] Dexamethasone has failed to show a benefit in preventing hospitalization or limiting length of stay after a single dose.[123] A reduction in duration of mechanical ventilation after IV dexamethasone has also not been proved.[124] In addition, a recent study of adults hospitalized with RSV found no significant difference in viral load or shedding duration in patients receiving 1 to 3 days of high-dose steroids.[125] Therefore, insufficient evidence exists for the use of steroids in patients with RSV bronchiolitis.[52,80]

In 2011, a review of the literature evaluating antibiotic use in bronchiolitis was published.[126] This review included 5 randomized controlled trials, 4 of which considered the use of macrolides in the treatment of bronchiolitis. Macrolides have added antiinflammatory properties that may address the inflammation that occurs with bronchiolitis. All but 1 study, with questionable bias, found no benefit to patient outcomes. Despite limited evidence, antibiotics continue to be highly prescribed for bronchiolitis without benefit of cure in children with RSV. For children with a suspicion of bacterial infection, use of a short course of antibiotics may be warranted until a pathogen is identified.[80] However, antibiotics have no role in changing the clinical course of viral disease and cannot be recommended for routine use.[43]

PATIENT AND FAMILY EDUCATION

For health care workers, educating parents is a priority.[64] Caregiver education starts on admission with an understandable explanation of the cause and effects of RSV and the expected clinical course for their child. Bronchiolitis can be a new and frightening experience to families and validating their concerns is important.[127] Explain to the family the many supportive management strategies are available for treatment of their child, despite there being no cure.

During hospitalization and after discharge, patients often require suctioning for increased nasal secretions. Although wall suction is often used in the hospital, parents do not have this option at home. Instruction on the use of a bulb syringe is helpful for caregivers and can make them more comfortable in caring for their child at home. Remind the parent to squeeze the bulb before gently inserting it into the child's nose. Nonmedicated saline drops may loosen mucus.[128] If a trial of bronchodilators is undertaken, some parents may confuse their child's condition with asthma. Explaining the difference between the two and why albuterol is being used for this select population may be helpful. In addition, parents often do not understand the absence of antibiotic treatment and other therapies. Explain that viruses cannot be cured with antibiotics, herbs, or other medicines. Parents may need to be reassured that their child's immune system is the main defense against the virus.[128,129]

As previously mentioned, hydration and nutrition are primary concerns in children with bronchiolitis. Nutrition is always a worry for parents. Explaining the details of nutrition delivery and giving parents opportunities to help where possible is important. On leaving the hospital, children may not show robust food and fluid intake. Therefore educating caregivers on the need to pay close attention to their child's intake and offering the child fluids is key to complete recovery.

Stressing the importance of prevention, including showing parents the correct hand washing technique, may reduce reinfection.[52] In an Italian study, only 12% of parents received advice about hand hygiene.[130] Parents were aware of transmission of germs via sneezing and coughing but were not as knowledgeable about the possibility of transmission from hands or other surfaces. Explain that smoking around a child increases the risk of respiratory illness, and eliminating exposure may help to prevent further complications of RSV bronchiolitis.[131] Avoiding exposure with sick children and young infants, keeping the child's surroundings clean, and washing toys regularly may also contribute to a quick recovery and prevent the spread of the disease.[132] For high-risk infants, help parents understand that palivizumab is safe and it must be repeated monthly during RSV season.[64]

After discharge, the child should follow up with the primary care provider (PCP) the week of discharge to make sure the child is improving. Explain that, for a few days or weeks, the child may not be at baseline and that reinfections are common.[13,133] Explain to the parent the signs and symptoms of worsening clinical condition, such as heavy breathing, grunting, nasal flaring, and retractions.[134] Instruct caregivers to continue taking the patient's temperature and to treat fevers as recommended by the provider. Remind parents to call their child's PCP if they ever are uncomfortable or have questions before the follow-up visit. Parents should call the PCP if the child is vomiting after most or all feeds, is having decreased intake, or has any of the following signs of dehydration: decreased wet diapers, crying without tears, and dry skin and mouth.[129] Reinforce the importance of seeking immediate medical attention if the child is working hard to breathe, runs a high fever, or develops a bluish color around lips or nail beds.

If your institution has information sheets on RSV and bronchiolitis, provide parents with these resources; if not, more information can be found on online resources such as the CDC,[7] MedLine Plus,[135] and the AAP.[131] The more information parents have, the better prepared they are to deal with situations that may arise.

SUMMARY

RSV is a highly infectious virus that commonly causes bronchiolitis and leads to high morbidity and a low, but important, incidence of mortality. Supportive therapy is the foundation of management. Hydration/nutrition and respiratory support including supplemental oxygen, hypertonic saline, and suctioning are important evidence-based interventions. For children with severe disease, CPAP or mechanical ventilation may be necessary therapeutic measures. Ribavirin is used rarely, for the treatment of patients with severe disease. Palivizumab provides important ongoing immunoprophylaxis during epidemic months for high-risk infants. Conventional chest physiotherapy, bronchodilators, steroids, and antibiotics do not have significant therapeutic benefit in the treatment of children with RSV bronchiolitis. Caregiver education and incorporating an explanation of all therapies and anticipatory guidance, including strategies for reducing the risk of infection, are vital.

REFERENCES

1. Nair H, Nokes D, Gessner BD, et al. Global burden of acute lower respiratory infectious due to respiratory syncytial virus in young children: a systematic review and meta-analysis. Lancet 2010;375:1545–55.
2. Shay DC, Holman RC, Newman RD, et al. Bronchiolitis associated hospitalizations among children 1980-1996. JAMA 1999;282:1440–6.
3. Walsh E. Respiratory syncytial virus infection in adults. Semin Respir Crit Care Med 2011;32:423–32.
4. Collins PL, Graham B. Viral and host factors in human respiratory syncytial virus pathogenesis. J Virol 2008;82:2040–55.
5. Stensballe L, Ravin H, Kristensen K, et al. Seasonal variation of maternally derived respiratory syncytial virus antibodies and association with infant hospitalizations for respiratory syncytial virus. J Pediatr 2009;154:296–8.
6. Bourgeois F, Valim C, McAdam A, et al. Relative impact of influenza and respiratory syncytial virus in young children. Pediatrics 2009;124:e1072–80.
7. Centers for Disease Control and Prevention. Respiratory syncytial virus infection (RSV). Available at: http://www.cdc.gov/rsv/index.html. Accessed April 30, 2012.
8. Brooks A, McBride JT, McConnochie MD, et al. Predicting deterioration in previously healthy infants hospitalized with respiratory syncytial virus infection. Pediatrics 1999;104:463–7.
9. Christakis DA, Cowan CA, Garrison MM, et al. Variation in inpatient testing and management of bronchiolitis. Pediatrics 2005;115:878–84.
10. Meerhoff T, Fleming D, Smith A, et al. Surveillance recommendations based on an exploratory analysis of respiratory syncytial virus reports derived from the European Influenza Surveillance System. BMC Infect Dis 2006;6:128.
11. Crowcroft N, Zambon M, Harrison T. Respiratory syncytial virus infection in infants admitted to paediatric intensive care units in London, and in their families. Eur J Pediatr 2008;167:395–9.
12. Hall C, Weinberg G, Iwane M, et al. The burden of respiratory syncytial virus infection in young children. N Engl J Med 2009;360:588–98.
13. Hurwitz J. Respiratory syncytial virus vaccine development. Expert Rev Vaccines 2011;10:1415–33.

14. Leader S, Kohlhase K. Respiratory syncytial virus-coded pediatric hospitalizations, 1997 to 1999. Pediatr Infect Dis J 2002;21:629–32.
15. Stang P, Brandenburg N, Carter B. The economic burden of respiratory syncytial virus-associated bronchiolitis hospitalizations. Arch Pediatr Adolesc Med 2001; 15:95–6.
16. Wright M, Piedimonte G. Respiratory syncytial virus prevention and therapy: past, present, and future. Pediatr Pulmonol 2011;46:324–47.
17. Li F, Zhu H, Sun R, et al. Natural killer cells are involved in acute lung immune injury caused by respiratory syncytial virus infection. J Virol 2012;86:2251–8.
18. McNamara P, Flanagan B, Selby A, et al. Pro- and anti-inflammatory responses in respiratory syncytial virus bronchiolitis. Eur Respir J 2004;23:106–12.
19. McNamara P, Flannagan B, Hart A, et al. Production of chemokines in the lungs of infants with severe respiratory syncytial virus bronchiolitis. J Infect Dis 2005; 19:1225–32.
20. Lindsley W, Blachere F, Davis K, et al. Distribution of airborne influenza virus and respiratory syncytial virus in an urgent care medical clinic. Clin Infect Dis 2010; 50:693–8.
21. Welliver R. The relationship of meteorological conditions to the epidemic activity in respiratory syncytial virus. Paediatr Respir Rev 2009;10:6–8.
22. Halstead DC, Jenkins SG. Continuous nonseasonal epidemic of respiratory syncytial virus infection in the southeast United States. South Med J 1998;91: 433–6.
23. Simoes E, Mutyara K, Soh S, et al. The epidemiology of respiratory syncytial virus lower respiratory tract infections in children less than 5 years of age in Indonesia. Pediatr Infect Dis J 2011;30:778–84.
24. Centers for Disease Control and Prevention. Respiratory syncytial virus infection: surveillance. Available at: www.cdc.gov/surveillance/nrevss/rsv/nat1-trend.html. Accessed May 2, 2012.
25. Eriksson M, Bennet R, Rotzen-Ostlund M, et al. Population-based rates of severe respiratory syncytial virus infection in children with and without risk factors, and outcome in a tertiary care setting. Acta Paediatr 2002;91:593–8.
26. Thorburn K, Kerr S, Taylor N. RSV outbreak in a paediatric intensive care unit. J Hosp Infect 2004;57:194–201.
27. Willson D, Landrigan C, Horn S, et al. Complications in infants hospitalized for bronchiolitis or respiratory syncytial virus pneumonia. J Pediatr 2003;143: S142–9.
28. Langley G, Anderson L. Epidemiology and prevention of respiratory syncytial virus infections among infants and young children. Pediatr Infect Dis J 2011; 30:510–7.
29. Duppenthaler A, Ammann R, Gorgievski-Hrisoho M, et al. Low incidence of respiratory syncytial virus hospitalisations in haemodynamically significant congenital heart disease. Arch Dis Child 2004;89:961–5.
30. Shi N, Palmer L, Chu B, et al. Association of RSV lower respiratory tract infection and subsequent healthcare use and costs: a Medicaid claims analysis in early preterm, later preterm and full term infants. J Med Econ 2011;14: 335–40.
31. Sampalis J. Morbidity and mortality after RSV-associated hospitalizations among premature Canadian infants. J Pediatr 2003;143:S150–6.
32. Zachariah P, Ruttenber M, Simoes E. Down syndrome and hospitalization due to respiratory syncytial virus: a population-based study. J Pediatr 2012;160: 827–31.

33. Welliver RC. Review of epidemiology and clinical risk factors for severe respiratory syncytial virus (RSV) infection. J Pediatr 2003;143:S112-7.
34. Wilkesmann A, Ammann R, Schildgen O, et al. Hospitalized children with respiratory syncytial virus infection and neuromuscular impairment face an increased risk of a complicated course. Pediatr Infect Dis J 2007;26:485-91.
35. Flores P, Rebelo-de-Andrade H, Goncalves P, et al. Bronchiolitis caused by respiratory syncytial virus in an area of Portugal: epidemiology, clinical features, and risk factors. Eur J Clin Microbiol Infect Dis 2004;23:39-45.
36. Lanari M, Giovannini M, Giuffre L, et al. Prevalence of respiratory syncytial virus infection in Italian infants hospitalized for acute lower respiratory tract infections, and association between respiratory syncytial virus infection risk factors and disease severity. Pediatr Pulmonol 2002;33:458-65.
37. Karr C, Lumley T, Schreuder A, et al. Effects of subchronic and chronic exposure to ambient air pollutants on infant bronchiolitis. Am J Epidemiol 2007;165:553-60.
38. Law B, Langley J, Allen U, et al. The Pediatric Investigators Collaborative Network on Infections in Canada study of predictors of hospitalization for respiratory syncytial virus infection for infants born at 33 through 35 completed weeks of gestation. Pediatr Infect Dis J 2004;23:806-14.
39. Koehoorn M, Karr C, Demers PA, et al. Descriptive Epidemiological features of bronchiolitis in a population-based cohort. Pediatrics 2008;122:1196-203.
40. Figueras-Aloy J, Carbonell-Estran X, Quero-Jimenez J, et al. FLIP-2 Study risk factors linked to respiratory syncytial virus infection requiring hospitalization in premature infants born in Spain at a gestational age of 32-35 weeks. Pediatr Infect Dis J 2008;27:788-93.
41. El Saleeby C, Bush A, Harrison L, et al. Respiratory syncytial virus load, viral dynamics, and disease severity in previously healthy naturally infected children. J Infect Dis 2011;204:996-1002.
42. Belderbos M, Houben M, Wilbrink B, et al. Cord blood vitamin D deficiency is associated with respiratory syncytial virus bronchiolitis. Pediatric 2011;127:e1513-20.
43. American Academy of Pediatrics. Respiratory syncytial virus. In: Pickering LK, Baker CJ, Kimberlin DW, editors. Red book: 2009 report of the Committee on Infectious Diseases. 28th edition. Elk Grove Village (IL): American Academy of Pediatrics; 2009. p. 560-9.
44. Karron R, Singleton R, Bulkow L, et al. Severe respiratory syncytial virus disease in Alaska native children. RSV Alaska Study Group. J Infect Dis 1999;180:41-9.
45. Miyair I, DeVincenzo JP. Human genetic factors and respiratory syncytial virus disease severity. Clin Microbiol Rev 2008;21:686-703.
46. Agency for Healthcare Research and Quality. Management of bronchiolitis in infants and children. Evidence report/technology assessment No. 69. Rockville (MD): Agency for Healthcare Research and Quality; 2003. AHRQ Publication No. 03-E014.
47. Thompson WW, Shay DK, Weintraub E, et al. Mortality associated with influenza and respiratory syncytial virus in the United States. JAMA 2003;289:179-86.
48. Levin D, Garg A, Hall L. A prospective randomized controlled blinded study of three bronchodilators in infants with respiratory syncytial virus bronchiolitis on mechanical ventilation. Pediatr Crit Care Med 2008;9:598-604.
49. Simoes E, Carbonell-Estrany X, Rieger C, et al. The effect of respiratory syncytial virus on subsequent recurrent wheezing in atopic and nonatopic children. J Allergy Clin Immunol 2010;126:256-62.

50. Jackson D, Lemanske R. The role of respiratory virus infections in childhood asthma inception. Immunol Allergy Clin North Am 2010;30:513–22.
51. Stensballe L, Simonsen J, Thomsen S, et al. The causal direction in the association between respiratory syncytial virus hospitalization and asthma. J Allergy Clin Immunol 2009;123:131–7.
52. Subcommittee on Diagnosis and Management of Bronchiolitis, American Academy of Pediatrics. Diagnosis and management of bronchiolitis. Pediatrics 2006;118:1774–93.
53. Leung A, Kellner J, Davies H. Respiratory syncytial virus bronchiolitis. JAMA 2005;97:1708–13.
54. Welliver R. RSV management: current and emerging treatments. Infect Dis Child 2012;(Suppl):12–6.
55. Mahony J. Detection of respiratory viruses by molecular methods. Clin Microbiol Rev 2008;21:716–47.
56. Falsey AR, Formica MA, Treanor J, et al. Comparison of quantitative reverse transcription-PCR to viral culture for assessment of respiratory syncytial virus shedding. J Clin Microbiol 2003;41:4160–5.
57. Wishaupt J, Russcher A, Smeets L, et al. Clinical impact of RT-PCR for pediatric acute respiratory infections: a controlled clinical trial. Pediatrics 2011;128:e1113–20.
58. Byington CL, Castillo H, Gerber K, et al. The effect of rapid respiratory viral diagnostic testing on antibiotic use in a children's hospital. Arch Pediatr Adolesc Med 2002;156:1230–4.
59. Heikkinen T, Valkonen H, Lehtonen L, et al. Hospital admission of high risk infants for respiratory syncytial virus infection: implications for palivizumab prophylaxis. Arch Dis Child Med-Fetal Neonatal Ed 2005;90:F64–8.
60. Aslanzadeh J, Zheng S, Li H, et al. Prospective evaluation of rapid antigen tests for diagnosis of respiratory syncytial virus and human metapneumovirus infections. J Clin Microbiol 2008;46:1682–5.
61. Casiano-Colon A, Hulbert B, Mayer J, et al. Lack of sensitivity of rapid antigen tests for diagnosis of respiratory syncytial virus infection in adults. J Clin Virol 2003;28:169–74.
62. Oosterheert JJ, van Loon A, Schuurman R, et al. Impact of rapid detection of viral and atypical bacterial pathogens by real-time polymerase chain reaction for patients with lower respiratory tract infection. Clin Infect Dis 2005;41:1438–44.
63. Freymuth F, Vabret A, Cuvillon-Nimal D, et al. Comparison of multiplex PCR assays and conventional techniques for the diagnostic of respiratory virus infections in children admitted to hospital with an acute respiratory illness. J Med Virol 2006;78:1488–504.
64. Wojtczak H. Strategies to increase adherence to RSV immunoprophylaxis. Infect Dis Child 2012;(Suppl):5–11.
65. Goodman G. RSV prevention and treatment: introduction and overview. Infect Dis Child 2012;(Suppl):3–4.
66. IMpact-RSV Study Group, Palivizumab, a humanized respiratory syncytial virus monoclonal antibody, reduces hospitalization from respiratory syncytial virus infection in high-risk infants. Pediatrics 1998;102:531–7.
67. Feltes TF, Cabalka A, Meissner H, et al. Palivizumab prophylaxis reduces hospitalization due to respiratory syncytial virus in young children with hemodynamically significant congenital heart disease. J Pediatr 2003;143:532–40.
68. Burls A, Sandercock J. Decision-making under conditions of uncertainty-what can we learn from palivizumab? Acta Paediatr 2011;100:1302–5.

69. Dizdar E, Aydemir C, Erdeve O, et al. Respiratory syncytial virus outbreak defined by rapid screening in a neonatal intensive care unit. J Hosp Infect 2010;75:292–4.

70. O'Connell K, Boo T, Keady D, et al. Use of palivizumab and infection control measures to control an outbreak of respiratory syncytial virus in a neonatal intensive care unit confirmed by real-time polymerase chain reaction. J Hosp Infect 2010;77:338–42.

71. Simoes E, Groothus J, Carbonell-Estrany X, et al. Palivizumab prophylaxis, respiratory syncytial virus, and subsequent recurrent wheezing. J Pediatr 2007;151:34–42.

72. Carbonell-Estrany X, Simoes E, Dagan R, et al. Motavizumab for prophylaxis of respiratory syncytial virus in high-risk children: a noninferiority trial. Pediatrics 2010;125:e31–51.

73. Feltes T, Sondheimer H, Tulloh R, et al. A randomized controlled trial of motavizumab versus palivizumab for the prophylaxis of serious respiratory syncytial virus disease in children with hemodynamically significant congenital heart disease. Pediatr Res 2011;70:186–91.

74. MedImmune. MedImmune discontinues development of motavizumab for RSV prophylaxis indication. Available at: http://pressroom.medimmune.com/press-releases/2010/12/21/medimmune-discontinues-development-of-motavizumab-for-rsv-prophylaxis-indication/. Accessed May 2, 2012.

75. Smart K, Paes B, Lanctot K. Changing costs and the impact on RSV prophylaxis. J Med Econ 2010;13:705–8.

76. Harris K, Anis A, Crosby M, et al. Economic evaluation of palivizumab in children with congenital heart disease: a Canadian perspective. Can J Cardiol 2011;27:e11–5.

77. Perrin K, Begue R. Use of palivizumab in primary practice. Pediatrics 2012;129:55–61.

78. Turner A, Begg C, Smith B, et al. The influence over a period of 8 years of patterns of prescribing palivizumab for patients with and without congenitally malformed hearts, and in admissions to paediatric intensive care. Cardiol Young 2009;19:346–51.

79. Frogel MP, Stewart DL, Hoopes M, et al. A systematic review of compliance with palivizumab administration for RSV immunoprophylaxis. J Manag Care Pharm 2010;16:46–58.

80. Zentz S. Care of infants and children with bronchiolitis: a systematic review. J Pediatr Nurs 2011;26:519–29.

81. Zorc J, Hall C. Bronchiolitis: recent evidence on diagnosis and management. Pediatrics 2010;125:342–9.

82. Simoes E, Carbonell-Estrany X, Fullarton, et al. European risk factors' model to predict hospitalization of premature infants born 33-35 weeks' gestational age with respiratory syncytial virus: validation with Italian data. J Matern-Fetal Neonatal Med 2011;24:152–7.

83. Black A, Brennan A. Breathing easy: implementing a bronchiolitis protocol. Pediatr Nurs 2011;37:129–35.

84. McDougall P. Caring for bronchiolitic infants needing continuous positive airway pressure. Pediatr Nurs 2011;23:30–6.

85. Cambonie G, Milesi C, Jaber S, et al. Nasal continuous positive airway pressure decreases respiratory muscles overload in young infants with severe acute viral bronchiolitis. Intensive Care Med 2008;34:1865–72.

86. Javouhey E, Barats A, Richard N. Noninvasive ventilation as primary ventilator support for infants with severe bronchiolitis. Intensive Care Med 2008;34:1608–14.

87. Thia L, McKenzie S, Blyth T. Randomized controlled trial of nasal continuous positive airways pressure (CPAP) in bronchiolitis. Arch Dis Child 2008;93:45–7.
88. Donlan M, Fontela P, Puligandla P. Use of continuous positive airway pressure (CPAP) in acute viral bronchiolitis: a systematic review. Pediatr Pulmonol 2011;46:736–46.
89. Greenough A. Role of ventilation in RSV disease: CPAP, ventilation, HFO, ECMO. Paediatr Respir Rev 2009;10(Suppl 1):26–8.
90. Essouri S, Duran P, Cheveret L. Optimal level of nasal continuous positive airway pressure in severe viral bronchiolitis. Intensive Care Med 2011;37:2002–7.
91. Papamoschou D. Theoretical validation of the respiratory benefits of helium-oxygen mixtures. Respir Physiol 1995;99:183–99.
92. Liet JM, Ducruet T, Gupta V, et al. Heliox inhalation therapy for bronchiolitis infants. Cochrane Database Syst Rev 2010;4:CD006915.
93. Martinon-Torres F, Rodriguez-Nunez A, Martino-Sanchez J, et al. Nasal continuous positive airway pressure with heliox versus air oxygen in infants with acute bronchiolitis: a crossover study. Pediatrics 2008;121:e1190–5.
94. Mayordomo-Colunga J. Helmet-delivered continuous positive airway pressure with heliox in respiratory syncytial virus bronchiolitis. Acta Paediatr 2010;99:308–11.
95. Cheifetz IM. Invasive and noninvasive pediatric mechanical ventilation. Respir Care 2003;48:442–53.
96. Mesiano G, Davis GM. Ventilatory strategies in the neonatal and paediatric intensive care units. Paediatr Respir Rev 2008;9:281–9.
97. Ventre K, Haroon M, Davison C. Surfactant therapy for bronchiolitis in critically ill infants. Cochrane Database Syst Rev 2006;3:CD005150.
98. Luo Z, Liu E, Luo J, et al. Nebulized hypertonic saline/salbutamol solution treatment in hospitalized children with mild to moderate bronchiolitis. Pediatr Int 2010;52:199–202.
99. Zhang L, Mendoza-Sassi R, Wainwright C, et al. Nebulized hypertonic saline solution for acute bronchiolitis in infants. Cochrane Database Syst Rev 2008;4:CD006458.
100. Kuzik B, Al-Qadhi S, Kent S, et al. Nebulized hypertonic saline in the treatment of viral bronchiolitis in infants. J Pediatr 2007;15:266–70.
101. Ventre K, Randolph A. Ribavirin for respiratory syncytial virus infection of the lower respiratory tract in infants and young children. Cochrane Database Syst Rev 2007;1:CD000181.
102. Ventre K, Randolph A. Withdrawn ribavirin for respiratory syncytial virus infection of the lower respiratory tract in infants and young children. Cochrane Database Syst Rev 2010;1:CD00181.
103. Glanville AR, Scott AI, Morton JM, et al. Intravenous ribavirin is a safe and cost-effective treatment for respiratory syncytial virus infection after lung transplantation. J Heart Lung Transplant 2005;24:2114–9.
104. Pelaez A, Lyon GM, Force SD, et al. Efficacy of oral ribavirin in lung transplant patients with respiratory syncytial virus lower respiratory tract infection. J Heart Lung Transplant 2009;28:67–71.
105. Mehta NM. Approach to enteral feeding in the PICU. Nutr Clin Pract 2009;24:377–87.
106. Joosten KF, Hulst JM. Prevalence of malnutrition in paediatric hospital patients. Curr Opin Pediatr 2008;20:590–6.
107. Zamberlan P, Delgad AF, Leone C, et al. Nutrition therapy in a pediatric intensive care unit: indications, monitoring and complication. J Parenter Enteral Nutr 2011;35:523–9.

108. Carcillo J. How should we nourish our sickest kids. JPEN J Parenter Enteral Nutr 2008;32:584–5.
109. Mehta N, McAleer D, Hamilton S, et al. Challenges to optimal enteral nutrition in multidisciplinary pediatric intensive care unit. JPEN J Parenter Enteral Nutr 2010;34:38–45.
110. Phipps L, Weber M, Ginder B, et al. A randomized controlled trial comparing three different techniques of nasojejunal feeding tube placement in critically ill children. JPEN J Parenter Enteral Nutr 2005;29:420–4.
111. Horn D, Chaboyer W. Gastric feeding in critically ill children: a randomized controlled trial. Am J Crit Care 2003;12:461–8.
112. Krohn K, Babl J, Reiter K, et al. Parenteral nutrition with standard solutions in paediatric intensive care patients. Clin Nutr 2005;24:274–80.
113. Hayden G. Bronchiolitis (acute): Chest physiotherapy for infants. Available at: http://connect.jbiconnectplus.org. Accessed May 1, 2012.
114. Perrotta C, Ortiz Z, Figuls M. Chest physiotherapy for acute bronchiolitis in pediatric patients between 0 and 24 months old. Cochrane Database Syst Rev 2007; 1:CD004873.
115. Postiaux G, Louis J, Labasse H, et al. Evaluation of an alternative chest physiotherapy method in infants with respiratory syncytial virus bronchiolitis. Respir Care 2011;56:989–94.
116. Gadomski A, Bhasale A. Bronchodilators for bronchiolitis. Cochrane Database Syst Rev 2006;3:CD001266.
117. Touzet S, Refabert L, Letrilliart L, et al. Impact of consensus development conference guidelines on primary care of bronchiolitis: are national guidelines being followed? J Eval Clin Pract 2007;13:651–6.
118. Hartling L, Bialy L, Milne A, et al. Steroids and bronchodilators for acute bronchiolitis in the first two years of life: systematic review and meta-analysis. BMJ 2011;342:d1714.
119. Amirav I, Luder A, Kruger N, et al. A double-blind, placebo-controlled, randomized trial of montelukast for acute bronchiolitis. Pediatrics 2008;122: e1249–55.
120. Bisgaard H, Flores-Nunez A, Goh A, et al. Study of montelukast for the treatment of respiratory symptoms of post-respiratory syncytial virus bronchiolitis in children. Am J Respir Crit Care Med 2008;178:854–60.
121. Kim C, Choi J, Kim H, et al. A randomized intervention of montelukast for post-bronchiolitis: effect on eosinophil degranulation. J Pediatr 2010;156: 749–54.
122. Blom D, Ermers M, Bont L, et al. Inhaled corticosteroids during acute bronchiolitis in the prevention of post-bronchiolitis wheezing. Cochrane Database Syst Rev 2007;1:CD004881.
123. Cornelli H, Zorc J, Mahajan P, et al. A multicenter, randomized, controlled trial of dexamethasone for bronchiolitis. N Engl J Med 2007;357:331–9.
124. Van Woensel J, Vyas H. Dexamethasone in children mechanically ventilated for lower respiratory tract infection cause by respiratory syncytial virus: a randomized controlled trail. Crit Care Med 2011;39:1779–83.
125. Lee F, Walsh E, Falsey AR. The effect of steroid use in hospitalized adults with respiratory syncytial virus-related illness. Chest 2011;140:1155–61.
126. Spurling GK, Donst J, Del Mar C, et al. Antibiotics for bronchiolitis in children. Cochrane Database Syst Rev 2011;6:CD005189.
127. Discenza D. Respiratory syncytial virus and the premature infant parent. Neonatal Netw 2011;30:345.

128. Moreno M. Advice for parents. Bronchiolitis and respiratory syncytial virus. Arch Pediatr Adolesc Med 2009;163:1072.

129. Punnoose A. Respiratory syncytial virus bronchiolitis. JAMA 2012;307:213.

130. DiCarlo P, Romano A, Plano M, et al. Children, parents and respiratory syncytial virus in Palermo, Italy: prevention is primary. J Child Health Care 2010;14: 396–407.

131. American Lung Association. Preventing bronchiolitis. Available at: http://www.lung.org/lung-disease/bronchiolitis/preventing-bronchiolitis.html. Accessed May 2, 2012.

132. Mayo Clinic Staff. Respiratory syncytial virus (RSV). Available at: http://www.mayoclinic.com/health/respiratory-syncytial-virus/DS00414. Accessed April 8, 2012.

133. Kemper A, Kennedy E, Dechert R, et al. Hospital readmission for bronchiolitis. Clin Pediatr 2005;44:509–13.

134. American Academy of Pediatrics. Bronchiolitis. 2011. Available at: http://www.healthychildren.org/English/health-issues/conditions/chest-lungs/Pages/Bronchiolitis.aspx. Accessed April 30, 2012.

135. Kaneshiro N. Bronchiolitis. Available at: http://www.nlm.nih.gov/medlineplus/ency/article/000975.htm. Accessed May 2, 2012.

A Review of Influenza
Implications for the Geriatric Population

Lori A. Dambaugh, BSN, RN, DNP-C[a,b],*

KEYWORDS

- Influenza • Geriatric • Pneumonia • Infection

KEY POINTS

- Influenza virus is a significant cause of morbidity and mortality in the United States.
- The ability of the influenza virus to shift and produce new strains is the reason new vaccines must be developed each year.
- The virus transmits easily from person to person, and is consequently a major health problem.
- High-risk populations for influenza include the geriatric population, pregnant women, immunosuppressed individuals, people with chronic illnesses, and those who live in close quarters.
- Vaccination is the single most effective way to prevent the spread of influenza.

HISTORY

Hippocrates was the first to report accounts of influenza-like illness.[1–5] The first recorded influenza pandemic was in 1510, and was reported to have spread from Europe throughout Asia and Africa.[5] The name influenza has its origins in the Italian language; in Italy it was thought that the disease was caused by the influence of the stars.[1] During the twentieth century influenza took an immense toll on the human population when more than 4 pandemics occurred: the Spanish Flu (1918–1919) is reported to have caused 50 million deaths, with the death toll reaching 500,000 in the United States alone, the Asian Flu (1957–1958) caused 60,000 deaths in the United States, the Hong Kong Flu (1968) claimed more than 40,000 in the United States, and the Russian Flu (1977) had relatively low mortality.[4]

The author has nothing to disclose.
[a] Progressive Pulmonary Care Unit, Rochester General Hospital, Department of Nursing, 1425 Portland Avenue, Rochester, NY 14617, USA; [b] St John Fisher College, Wegmans School of Nursing, 3690 East Avenue, Rochester 14618, New York, USA
* St John Fisher College, Wegmans School of Nursing, 3690 East Avenue, Rochester 14618, New York, USA.
E-mail address: lori.dambaugh@rochestergeneral.org

Crit Care Nurs Clin N Am 24 (2012) 573–580
http://dx.doi.org/10.1016/j.ccell.2012.07.005
0899-5885/12/$ – see front matter © 2012 Elsevier Inc. All rights reserved.

SEASONALITY

Unlike other viruses, influenza follows a typical seasonal pattern. Annual epidemics of influenza in the United States usually occur during fall and winter. In the Northern hemisphere most cases of influenza are seen between the months of October and March; conversely, influenza is seen in the Southern Hemisphere between the months of May and October.[6] The rationale for the peak of influenza during winter months is poorly understood, but several theories exist to explain this phenomenon. One theory postulates that flu is more common in the winter months when people have a tendency to assemble in enclosed and often poorly ventilated environments.[7] Another theory is that the stability of the virus may be improved by cooler temperatures.[8] Host immunity may be diminished during cold weather.[8] Vitamin D deficiency in the winter months may reduce effectiveness of the innate immune system.[8]

EPIDEMIOLOGY

Influenza viruses are single-stranded RNA viruses that belong to the family Orthomyxoviridae and are classified as types A, B, or C.[5,8] Type A influenza viruses are the most prevalent and typically the most virulent. Type A outbreaks typically have an abrupt onset, then peak over 2 to 3 weeks and last for approximately 2 to 3 months. Influenza A viruses are categorized into subtypes based on 2 surface antigens, hemagglutinin (HA) and neuraminidase (NA).[9] Four HA subtypes (H1, H2, H3, and H5) and 2 NA subtypes (N1 and N2) are known to affect humans.[2] HA enables the virus to penetrate the cells in the respiratory tract, and NA helps facilitate movement from the host cell to infect new cells in the respiratory tract.[6]

Influenza B viruses are usually less virulent and less likely to cause epidemics. Influenza B viruses are typically found in humans, but have been isolated from pigs and seals.[5] Neither influenza B nor influenza C viruses are subtyped in the same manner as influenza A viruses. Recently, 2 distinct genetic lineages of B viruses have been identified: Yamagata and Victoria.[2,9] Influenza C viruses can cause mild illness in humans; however, they do not have the capacity to cause epidemics or pandemics.

The ability of the influenza virus to shift and produce new strains is the reason new vaccines must be developed each year. Influenza viruses undergo frequent spontaneous mutations in their surface proteins. Antigenic drift is a term that points to the slight mutations that take place in the HA and NA proteins of the virus.[6] Influenza A is known to drift more than influenza B. These drifting strains of influenza are the basis of the need for new influenza vaccine each year. Outbreaks that occur as a result of antigenic drift are usually less severe than those that occur with antigenic shifts. Antigenic shift occurs when major changes take place in the HA or NA proteins; however, they occur less frequently than antigenic drifts. Influenza A viruses are the only type of influenza virus that undergo antigenic shift, and are the major causes of epidemics or pandemics.[6,9]

TRANSMISSION

The influenza virus is thought to be highly contagious and spreads easily from person to person, although experts differ in opinion concerning the precise mechanism of transmission. It is generally thought that the flu virus is spread by large-particle respiratory transmission dispersed by coughing or sneezing near a susceptible person.[9] These droplets may then be deposited on to the mucosal surface of the susceptible person's upper respiratory tract.[5] Transmission is thought to occur at close range rather than longer distances, because droplets do not remain suspended in air for long periods of time.[1,9] There is less evidence of transmission from environmental surfaces, although it is thought that if viruses land on hard surfaces they can survive for 24 hours, and have the potential to infect individuals who touch that surface and then transfer it from their hands to their mouth or nose.[6] The incubation period is 1 to 4 days with average incubation of 2 days, and the virus may be transmitted a day before onset of symptoms and continue for up to 5 to 10 days.[2,9] Severely immunocompromised patients may shed virus for weeks or months.[5,9] Proper hand hygiene and avoidance of close contact with those with flulike symptoms are prudent recommendations to halt transmission. Those at highest risk are individuals who are residing in closed environments, such as assisted living or nursing homes and hospitals, which are disproportionately represented by individuals aged 65 years and older.

SIGNS AND SYMPTOMS

Influenza is an acute viral illness characterized by an abrupt onset of fever, sore throat, headache, nonproductive cough, rhinitis, myalgia, and generalized malaise.[9,10] Despite the fact that the influenza virus replicates in the respiratory epithelium, respiratory symptoms are not always the most prominent feature of infection. Myalgias are very common presenting symptoms of influenza, but the reason for this is not well understood. It is thought that the infection with the virus possibly triggers the release of cytokines as part of the immune response, which then may be responsible for the neuromuscular symptoms.[1]

In uncomplicated cases of influenza, symptoms last for approximately 5 days; however, 20% of individuals may experience symptoms for longer than 10 days.[1,10] Complications can occur from influenza, especially in those age 65 and older and patients with preexisting chronic conditions. Complications from influenza include viral pneumonia, exacerbation of preexisting cardiac or pulmonary conditions, secondary bacterial pneumonia, sinusitis, and possible secondary infection with other viral or bacterial pathogens.[11] Influenza A may manifest with severe headache and generalized malaise. Patients infected with influenza B may experience nausea, vomiting, and diarrhea as more prominent symptoms.

The classic symptom of pyrexia may not be seen in the geriatric population, owing to an aging immune system or immunosenescence. Immunosenescence is defined as the progressive age-associated alterations that occur in the immune system.[12] Diagnosis and treatment of influenza is particularly important in this population, because of their vulnerability to secondary infections such as pneumonia and respiratory syncytial virus (RSV).

DIAGNOSIS

Diagnostic testing of individuals is not usually required because diagnosis can typically be made on the basis of clinical history and typical signs and symptoms of influenza, especially during seasonal outbreaks. Laboratory tests are fairly expensive and typically do not affect the management or progression of the infection.[6] However, diagnostic testing is appropriate in several circumstances. During large outbreaks diagnostic testing is essential for surveillance of the disease, differentiation of the virus and its subtypes, and clinical confirmation.[2] Diagnostic confirmation and identification of influenza during large public outbreaks allows public health agencies to establish which strains of virus and subtypes are in circulation.[1] The Centers for Disease Control and Prevention (CDC) also recommends diagnostic confirmation for hospitalized patients and for individuals when a positive influenza diagnosis would necessitate a change in the course of clinical management, affect patients' close contacts, or have implications for infection control.[2] In individuals 65 years and older, diagnostic confirmation may be important because a decrease in the usual immune response, fever, and common symptoms may not be seen in this population. Influenza in the older population may present as a change in usual behavior patterns, restlessness, or respiratory symptoms. Thus diagnostic testing may be important during large seasonal outbreaks.

There are multiple diagnostic testing options for influenza; however, each vary in their ability to identify virus types and subtypes. Rapid Influenza Diagnostic Testing (RIDT) is an immunoassay that identifies the presence of influenza A and B viral nucleoprotein antigens present in respiratory specimens.[11] Acceptable specimens include nasal pharyngeal swab, nasal wash, and nasal aspirate. Results are reported as positive or negative, but may not provide information on subtypes or strains of virus, although some RIDTs are able to differentiate between A and B virus.[2,11] Results can generally be available in less than 30 minutes.[2] The disadvantage to this type of testing is that during periods of low influenza activity, false-positive results may occur even though the tests have high specificity.[11] Negative results do not exclude infection with influenza virus in individuals, and if influenza is still suspected, further testing should occur. Further testing should also occur if a patient tests positive by RIDT and influenza prevalence in the community is low, a false-positive result is suspected, or a patient has recent exposure to animals such as pigs and poultry, which could possibly transmit a novel influenza A virus.[7] Further testing can include viral culture, immunofluorescence, or reverse transcriptase–polymerase chain reaction.

Viral cultures have been the gold standard for identification of influenza virus. Acceptable specimens for viral cultures are nasopharyngeal swab, nasopharyngeal or bronchial wash, nasal or endotracheal aspirate, and sputum, which usually take 3 to 10 days to process.[11] Viral cultures are highly specific and sensitive.[2] Viral cultures have the ability to differentiate between different strains and subtypes of virus. Despite their high degree of sensitivity and specificity, viral cultures may not be useful in treatment decisions because of their long processing time. However, diagnosis by viral culture is important for surveillance of new strains and in the monitoring of antiviral resistance.[11]

The polymerase chain reaction (PCR) is a highly sensitive test (86%–100%).[11] The PCR test takes anywhere from 1 to 5 hours to perform, and acceptable specimens are the same as those collected for viral culture.[11] The PCR test is able to identify influenza virus by using nucleic acid that is extracted from the specimens. Immunofluorescence assays are processed in 1 to 4 hours, and specimens can include nasopharyngeal swab, bronchial wash, and nasal and endotracheal aspirate.[11] Serology testing is not recommended by the CDC to provide individual-level clinical decision making. Serology testing is not widely available and is generally used for public health investigations.[11]

TREATMENT

In most individuals influenza is an illness for which treatment is limited to rest and symptom management. Despite the fact that influenza is usually self limiting, individuals who are 65 years and older and have preexisting conditions such as heart disease, respiratory disease, and diabetes are more susceptible to developing secondary complications such as pneumonia. These high-risk individuals may require antiviral treatment and, possibly, hospitalization to treat complications. The treatment of viral infections is difficult owing to several factors. Viruses are very minute intracellular parasites, which are difficult for antiviral drugs to attack. Viral drugs often have toxic side effects. Viral infections are usually fully established before symptoms appear and diagnosis is established.[1] To be effective and shorten the course of the illness, antiviral drug therapy should preferably be implemented within 48 hours of symptom onset.[1,2]

There are 4 approved antiviral agents available in the United States: amantadine, rimantadine, zanamivir, and oseltamivir. Zanamivir and oseltamivir are antiviral medications classified as neuraminidase inhibitors, and both are active against influenza A and B viruses.[13] During the 2011 influenza season, zanamivir and oseltamivir were the recommended antivirals for the treatment of flu.[13] The usual duration of treatment is 5 days, although longer treatment courses may be deemed appropriate for patients who are still severely ill after the 5-day course.[13] Zanamivir is not recommended for patients with chronic obstructive pulmonary disease (COPD) or asthma, and cautious use is advised in the geriatric population.[2] Amantadine and rimantadine are related antivirals classified as adamantanes. Adamantanes are active against influenza A virus but not influenza B virus. The CDC reports that resistance to adamantanes by the influenza A (H3N2) and the 2009 H1N1 viruses has been developing.[13] Resulting secondary bacterial infections should be treated with judicious use of appropriate antibiotics.

VACCINATION

Vaccination is the most effective public health measure to help prevent infection with the influenza virus.[14] Efficacy with the influenza vaccine is approximately 70% to 80% in healthy adults when the vaccine closely matches the circulating strains.[6] There are currently 2 types of vaccines that are effective in preventing the influenza virus: trivalent inactivated influenza vaccine (TIV) and live attenuated influenza vaccine (LAIV). TIV and LAIV are both widely available in the United States. TIV contains inactivated viruses that are antigenically equivalent to the annual recommended strains.[14] Because TIV is a killed virus, it is unable to cause influenza. TIV is recommended for individuals older than 6 months, and can be given to both healthy people and individuals with chronic medical conditions. In adults the TIV vaccine is administered via the intramuscular route in the deltoid muscle. The most frequent side effect of vaccination is a mild local reaction such as redness or swelling at the injection site.[10] Systemic side effects such as myalgias, low-grade fever, or headaches have also been reported.[6] Studies have demonstrated that systemic symptoms are usually no higher than those rates seen with placebo injections.[10] Contraindications to vaccination with TIV include an allergy to eggs, acute febrile illness, and Guillain-Barré syndrome within 6 weeks of a prior influenza vaccination.[14]

LAIV is a live attenuated virus administered by the intranasal route. LAIV does not contain thimerosal, a preservative used to reduce bacterial growth in vaccines. LAIV should not be given to individuals with risk factors for influenza-related complications.[14] LAIV is not recommended for individuals younger than 2 or older than 49 years.[14] Side effects of LAIV may include mild temperature elevation and nasal congestion. Systemic symptoms commonly seen with influenza are rare.

The World Health Organization publishes recommendations on the strains that are expected to cause seasonal influenza. The 3 most virulent strains in circulation are identified and recommended for inclusion in the vaccine for the current year to afford protection against the strains thought likely to cause epidemics in that particular year.[7] Approximately 80% of the time there is a suitable match between influenza strains and circulating viruses each season.[10]

Although there has been increased attention and education afforded to the influenza vaccine in recent years, there remains resistance in the general public to receiving the vaccine. Individuals who are likely to avoid vaccination include those who think they are in good health, have not received advice from a nurse or doctor, perceive they are not at risk for infection, or maintain negative views about the safety and efficacy of the vaccine.[1] It is important for health care providers to dispel the many commonly held myths related to the influenza vaccine. One common fallacy is that receiving the influenza vaccine may infect an individual with the flu virus. Health care providers are in a position to explain the risks and benefits of the influenza vaccine to alleviate this common fear. Another common myth is that despite receiving the influenza vaccine, individuals still become infected with the influenza virus. This reasoning may be due to the patient's perception of the common cold being analogous with flu, or during a season when a flu strain is in circulation that was not included in the vaccine.[6] Education by health care providers is an important component in any vaccination campaign to help improve rates of immunization.

VACCINE CONSIDERATIONS FOR OLDER INDIVIDUALS

Influenza is a significant seasonal infection that is related to considerable morbidity and mortality, and the geriatric population is at high risk for serious complications that often result in hospitalizations. The vulnerability of the geriatric population has made this a high-priority group for routine vaccination. Vaccinations for individuals older than 65 years have been associated with substantial reductions in hospitalizations for influenza-related complications, including pneumonia.[10] In adults older than 65 years there may be a reduced immune response to vaccination; however, there is little evidence in support of this theory.[14] It is postulated that infection after vaccination is more likely the result of the age-related inability to respond to the vaccination.[14] Studies have reported that influenza vaccination may reduce winter mortality risk from any cause by 50% among the geriatric population.[15] Benefits of vaccination for this population include decreased hospitalization for pneumonia and other influenza-related conditions.

CASE STUDY

Joan is an 82-year-old woman who complained of progressive muscle soreness, fatigue, and slight dyspnea over 3 days. Joan lived independently in a senior housing community and had a history of COPD and type 2 diabetes. Joan was a former smoker and quit more than 20 years ago. She used 2 L oxygen via nasal cannula at baseline. Joan received the influenza vaccine last year and complained of developing flulike symptoms immediately after vaccination. This year, despite extensive education from her health care provider about the importance of yearly vaccination, she refused vaccination.

On day 4 of Joan's symptoms, she was visited by her son who observed that she was noticeably dyspneic. Her son called emergency medical services, and she was brought by ambulance to her local emergency department (ED). On arrival, she was febrile at 37.3°C (99.1°F), with stable vital signs with labored respirations, and her oxygen saturation was 86% on 2 L of oxygen. Initial ED management included 1 L 0.9% normal saline at 125 mL/h, chest radiograph, 2 albuterol nebulizers, 2 sets of blood cultures, and a flu culture. Her oxygen was titrated up to 5 L via nasal cannula. Joan was diagnosed with community-acquired pneumonia and was started on antibiotics. She was transferred to the medical unit for monitoring, hydration, oxygen, and intravenous antibiotics.

One hour after transfer to the medial surgical unit, Joan was noted by her nurse to be having increased respiratory distress; her oxygen saturation decreased to 82% on 5 L of oxygen. An arterial blood gas was drawn demonstrated respiratory acidosis. Joan was emergently intubated in response to the respiratory failure, and transferred to the intensive care unit. The rapid flu was confirmed positive. Joan was started on the antiviral oseltamivir. Despite aggressive treatment, Joan became hemodynamically unstable, demonstrating signs of severe sepsis. She died of the complications of sepsis and multiple organ failure.

This case illustrates the importance of annual vaccination in the geriatric population, which is at high risk for developing serious complications related to infection with the influenza virus. This case also demonstrates the need for careful consideration of influenza diagnosis in the geriatric population, because of the possibility of an atypical presentation of flu not characterized by an abrupt onset of fever. Cautious deliberation must be given to individuals older than 65 who present with nonspecific symptoms during the flu season, to ensure prompt diagnosis and timely treatment.

SUMMARY

The influenza virus is a significant cause of morbidity and mortality each year in the United States. Infection with the influenza virus in healthy individuals is certainly an unpleasant experience; however, in individuals aged 65 years and older infection is serious and may lead to complications, hospitalization, and death. Prompt diagnosis and treatment is imperative for individuals 65 years and older. Vaccination is an effective tool for prevention of influenza infection and is of particular importance in the geriatric population.

REFERENCES

1. Gould D. The challenges of caring for patients with influenza. Nurs Older People 2011;23(10):28–34.
2. Kung YM. A close up view of flu. Nurse Pract 2010;35:47–52.
3. Taubenberger J, Morens D. The pathology of influenza virus infections. Annu Rev Pathol 2008;3:499–522.
4. Nanumona E, Parisi S, Castronovo D, et al. Pneumonia and influenza hospitalizations in elderly people with dementia. J Am Geriatr Soc 2009;57:2192–9.
5. Association of Operating Room Nurses. AORN guidance statements: human and avian influenza and severe acute respiratory syndrome. AORN J 2006;84:284–98.
6. Wilcox A. Influenza: epidemiology and prevention. Pract Nurs 2011;22:538–43.
7. Ward L, Draper J. A review of the factors involved in older people's decision making with regard to influenza vaccination: a literature review. J Clin Nurs 2007;17:5–16.
8. Nelson M, Holmes E. The evolution of epidemic influenza. Nature 2007;8: 196–205.
9. Centers for Disease Control, Prevention. Prevention and control of influenza: recommendations of the advisory committee on immunization practices 2008. MMWR Recomm Rep 2008;57:1–59.
10. Nichol K. Influenza vaccination in the elderly. Drugs Aging 2005;22:495–515.
11. Centers for Disease Control and Prevention, National Center for Immunization and Respiratory Disease. Influenza symptoms and the role of laboratory diagnostics. 2011. Available at: http://www.cdc.gov/flu/professionals/diagnosis/labroles procedures.htm. Accessed January 1, 2011.
12. Aw D, Silva A, Palmer D. Immunosenescence: emerging challenges for an ageing population. Immunology 2007;120:435–46.
13. Centers for Disease Control and Prevention, National Center for Immunization and Respiratory Diseases. 2011–2012 influenza antiviral medications: summary for clinicians. 2011. Available at: http://www.cdc.gov/flu/professionals/antivirals/ summary-clinicians.htm. Accessed February 1, 2012.

14. Centers for Disease Control, Prevention. Prevention and control of influenza with vaccines: recommendations of the advisory committee on immunization practices 2010. MMWR 2010;59:1–61.
15. Simonsen L, Reichert T, Viboud C, et al. Impact of influenza vaccination on seasonal mortality in the U.S. elderly population. Arch Intern Med 2005;165: 265–72.

Critical Care for Frostbite

Teri Lynn Kiss, RN, MS, MSSW, CCRN

KEYWORDS

- Frostbite • Cold injury • Rewarming • Risk factors • Prevention

KEY POINTS

- Frostbite occurs when the skin temperature cools to below 0°C with the formation of extracellular ice crystals.
- Injury severity depends on temperature, duration of exposure, and the amount and depth of frozen tissue.
- The mainstays of treatment are rapid rewarming and watchful waiting.
- With rewarming, an inflammatory response develops, contributing to ischemia and tissue loss.

INTRODUCTION

Cold injuries are divided into 3 categories: freezing injuries, nonfreezing injuries, and hypothermia. Frostbite is the condition whereby damage to skin and other tissue occurs as a result of freezing, and is a preventable injury.[1] Frostbite is a concern for those who live, work, and play in polar and other cold-weather regions. The hazardous environment necessitates the awareness of the potentials for injury related to extreme cold weather, and the knowledge and skills to prevent injury from occurring. Daily activities related to commuting to work, occupations, lifestyles or life situations that require being outside in freezing temperatures, and leisure-time activities that involve prolonged exposure times become opportunities for frostbite to develop.

The military experience with frostbite is well documented. Xenophon, in 400 BC, led an army of Greek soldiers through the mountains of Armenia where they experienced severe cold weather, resulting in amputations from frostbite and death by exposure. Baron Dominique-Jean Larrey, Napoleon's surgeon-in-chief, provided the first detailed description of the management of frostbite based on his observations of frostbite injury occurring during the Russian retreat in the winter of 1812.[2–4] The United States military have suffered casualties related to cold injury, including frostbite, with a majority occurring during World War II.[3,5]

The author has nothing to disclose.

Medical Unit 2 South, Fairbanks Memorial Hospital, 1650 Cowles Street, Fairbanks, AK 99701, USA

E-mail address: tlynnkiss@gmail.com

Crit Care Nurs Clin N Am 24 (2012) 581–591

http://dx.doi.org/10.1016/j.ccell.2012.07.001   **ccnursing.theclinics.com**

Civilian cases have increased over the years, in part because of increases in social issues such as homelessness, but also because of greater participation in winter sports. The spectrum of injury can range from minimal tissue loss to extensive necrosis necessitating amputation. Long-term sequelae can include chronic pain, sensitivity to cold, and a predisposition to cold injury in the future.[6–8]

EPIDEMIOLOGY

The incidence of frostbite is difficult to ascertain, as hospital data generally represent the most severe cases.[7] There are estimates of 4800 cases of frostbite each year in the United States.[9] People living in northern latitudes have an especially high incidence of frostbite, with one study of 6000 Finnish men showing 44% had sustained some degree of frostbite at least once.[7] The Alaska Trauma Registry lists hypothermia and frostbite as one of the top 10 causes of nonfatal hospitalized injuries for Alaska residents in the years 2001 to 2010.[10]

Historical data show the US Military experienced casualties from cold injury, with approximately 2000 from World War I, 91,000 from World War II, and 6300 from the Korean War. The Afghanistan Conflict, the first large-scale conflict in a cold-weather region since the Korean Conflict, had only 2 cases of frostbite identified. Advances in types of cold-weather gear, education, and training with acclimation of military personnel to cold weather may account for this difference.[5] Between 1990 and 1995, first- and second-degree frostbite accounted for 99.3% of reported cases of cold-weather injury among US soldiers in Alaska, with male African American soldiers significantly more susceptible than Caucasian soldiers.[11] The period 1996 to 2011 showed a slight decrease in the rate of frostbite but consistently demonstrated the highest rates in females, in those younger than 20 years, and in black, non-Hispanic soldiers.[12–14]

Factors associated with frostbite (**Table 1**) include environmental, individual, behavioral, health related, certain medications, situational, and others.[1,6,8,15,16] Mohr and colleagues[17] characterize factors as the I's of frostbite: intoxicated, incompetent, infirm, insensate, inducted (increased risk during war time), inexperience, and indigent.

Deep frostbite injuries that require hospitalization are usually of the hands and feet. Most minor injuries are superficial and affect the face and head, including the nose, chin, earlobes, cheeks, and lips. Other affected areas include the buttocks and penis.[6–8]

PATHOPHYSIOLOGY

Frostbite occurs when tissue temperatures fall below 0°C, a temperature slightly below the freezing point of water, because of the electrolyte content of cells and extracellular fluid. Wet skin cools faster, will reach a lower temperature, and will freeze at a higher threshold.[7,15] Air temperature, wind speed, and wetness are determinants of heat loss. At temperatures below −10°C (14°F), wind speed increases the risk of injury from cold. The wind-chill temperature (WCT) index estimates the cooling power of the environment and indicates frostbite times for exposed facial skin in minutes. At −37°C (−35°F) with a wind speed of 8 km/h (5 mph), frostbite could occur in 30 minutes (**Fig. 1**).[18]

The severity and degree of tissue injury are related to temperature and duration of exposure, with duration being the more significant factor.[16,19] The continuum of injury ranges from irreversible cellular destruction to reversible changes occurring after rewarming. Two mechanisms for tissue injury have been identified: cellular death

Table 1
Factors of frostbite

Environment	Individual	Behavioral	Physiologic	Situational	Other
Temperature	Physical characteristics	Alcohol use	Peripheral vascular diseases	Homelessness	Trauma resulting in immobilizing injury or compromise to distal circulation
Wind	Age	Dehydration	Peripheral or autonomic neuropathy	Lack of heat source	
Wetness	Gender	Fatigue	Endocrine conditions	Transportation breakdown	
Duration of cold exposure	Genetic susceptibility	Smoking	Hyperhidrosis		
Contact with cold objects or liquids		Inappropriate or inadequate garments	Prior cold injury		
High altitude (>17000 feet)		Constrictive clothing	Psychiatric disorder		
Latitude of residence (annual no. of cold days)		Prolonged stationary posture	Altered mental status		
		Use of protective ointments	Hypoxia		
		Situational misjudgment	Hypothermia		
			Medications (β-Blockers), (Sedatives Neuroleptics), (α-Adrenergic blockers)		

Data from Refs. [1,6–8,15,16]

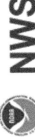

Fig. 1. National Weather Service wind-chill chart. (*Courtesy of* NOAA, National Weather Service. Available at: http://www.nws.noaa.gov/os/windchill/index.shtml.)

occurring at time of exposure to cold, and the deterioration and necrosis from progressive ischemia.[19]

Local cold injury happens through a succession of changes divided into phases that may overlap: prefreeze, freeze-thaw, vascular stasis, and progressive or late ischemic.[8,16,20] During the prefreeze phase, cutaneous blood flow is affected and vasoconstriction occurs. In the freeze-thaw phase there is alternating vasodilation and vasoconstriction. During the freeze phase, ice crystals form in the extracellular space causing intracellular dehydration and hyperosmolality. The thaw phase is when the vasodilation that occurs reestablishes blood flow, resulting in thrombosis. The vascular stasis phase is characterized by circulatory shunting between the injured and noninjured margins causing stasis, coagulation, and thrombus formation. The late ischemic phase includes thrombus-induced inflammation, hypoxia, and necrosis.[16,19,20]

Initial injury comes from the extracellular formation of ice crystals, causing direct damage to the cell membrane. As freezing continues, microvascular function is compromised, intracellular ice crystals form, and irreversible damage or death may occur. The body responds to cooling by alternating cycles of vasodilation and vasoconstriction, known as the hunting response or cold-induced vasodilation, a warming mechanism for affected areas that continues until the core temperature is threatened.[16,19] During rewarming, reperfusion injury occurs involving oxygen free radicals, neutrophil activation, prostaglandins and thromboxane, and other inflammatory changes. Once the hunting response stops, uncycled vasoconstriction continues, resulting in progressive hypoxia, ischemia, thrombosis, and tissue necrosis.[7,8,16,19]

The progressive ischemic damage seen in frostbite is similar to damage in thermal burn injury. The difference is in the extent of microcirculatory damage and recovery in frostbite, with the inflammatory process lasting longer than in burns and angiogenesis occurring more rapidly in frostbite.[21] The role of inflammatory mediators, including prostaglandins and thromboxanes, bradykinin, and histamine, in edema formation, endothelial injury, and interruption of dermal blood flow is supported in burn models; the discovery of thromboxane and prostaglandin in frostbite blister fluid points to the role of inflammatory mediators in frostbite.[19]

CLINICAL PRESENTATION

Frostnip is distinct from frostbite, and is a superficial nonfreezing cold injury associated with vasoconstriction on exposed skin with frost forming on the surface, with resultant numbness and pallor. The symptoms resolve quickly with warming techniques, and no long-term damage occurs. The appearance of frostnip signals conditions favorable for frostbite to occur.[20]

The initial symptoms of frostbite are generally described as a cold numbness and, possibly, some pain. Continued freezing produces paresthesia and/or numbness, with some areas of blanching blending into uninjured skin. Clumsiness and a loss of fine motor control (in the hands) may also occur. Later features include white and waxy skin with distinct margins from uninjured tissue and a wooden feeling in the affected area. Rewarming is often painful and includes feelings of burning, aching, sharp pain, and decreased sensation.[6,8,15,19]

Frostbite has been historically classified into 4 degrees following the scheme for thermal burn injury. A simplified classification of superficial and deep was proposed by Mills and Whaley.[22] True frostbite injuries appear similar at initial presentation. The classification of frostbite is applied after rewarming.[19]

First-degree frostbite is characterized by insensate white areas, edema, and hyperemia without the presence of blisters. Second-degree frostbite is characterized by the presence of clear blisters, erythema, and edema. First and second degrees are classified as superficial frostbite with the injury limited to skin and subcutaneous tissue that remains pliable, reversible neurovascular dysfunction, and minimal to no tissue loss. Third-degree frostbite is full-thickness skin and subcutaneous freezing with hemorrhagic blisters and skin necrosis. Fourth-degree frostbite is full-thickness skin, subcutaneous tissue, muscle, tendon, and bone damage. Third and fourth degrees are classified as deep frostbite with the dermis being nonpliable, the injured tissue remaining mottled and insensate even after rewarming, and tissue loss being inevitable (**Table 2**).[6,8,20,22–24]

The classification scheme describes wound conditions, but does not necessarily correlate with the clinical outcome. Cauchy[25] proposed a predictive classification system based on the findings after initial rewarming and then on day 2. The parameters involve the radiotracer uptake on bone scan and the presence of blisters. The classification ranges from Grade 1 (no amputation, no long-term sequelae) to Grade 4 (amputation, possible development of thrombosis or sepsis, functional sequelae).[25]

Favorable prognostic indicators for recovery include intact sensation, normal skin color, and clear filled blisters. Less favorable indicators include dark fluid-filled blisters, mottled skin with nonblanching cyanosis, and hard, nondeforming skin.[19]

CARE OF FROSTBITE INJURY

Larrey's observations of frostbite injuries during the Russian retreat of 1812 prompted recommendations of slow rewarming by rubbing the affected part with snow, avoiding using the heat from fire to rewarm the affected part because it caused congelation, and considering amputation as a treatment of last resort.[2–4] His recommendation against rapid rewarming influenced treatment of frostbite well into the twentieth century.[3] In World War I, the American Military Manual recommended rubbing the frozen part with wet snow or ice water. Soviet scientists had been studying rapid rewarming in the 1930s, although this was unknown to Western scientists. In the 1940s, Fuhrman and Crismon used the information in their research and published an article describing rapid rewarming that changed the ideas on the best method of frostbite treatment.[26]

Research on frostbite was intensified in the 1950s and 1960s, based on the fear of war with the Soviet Union and the need for fighting in cold environments. Meryman and others demonstrated that the rate of freezing influenced the size of ice crystals, with slower freezing producing larger crystals.[26] Hamill's use of rapid rewarming

Table 2 Stages of frostbite			
First Degree	**Second Degree**	**Third Degree**	**Fourth Degree**
Superficial		**Deep**	
Partial skin freezing	Full-thickness skin freezing	Freezing of skin and subcutaneous tissue	Freezing of skin, subcutaneous tissue, muscle, tendon, and bone
No blisters	Blisters with clear or milky fluid	Hemorrhagic blisters; some tissue necrosis	Large amount of tissue necrosis
Erythema or hyperemia	Erythema	Cyanosis or dark red nonblanchable skin	Deep red and mottled skin
No or minor edema	Edema	Edema	Little or no edema

Data from Refs.[6,8,20,22–24]

prompted further clinical investigation in Alaska by Mills and colleagues,[4,20,23,26] resulting in guidelines for frostbite care that have changed little through the years. The goals of management are tissue salvage, maximal return of function, optimized nutrition for healing, and prevention of complications.

The care of frostbite injury is generally characterized as prethaw field care, rewarming, and post-thaw care.[19,20,23] Field care is generally limited to protecting the frozen tissue from further damage. A primary focus is preventing refreezing injury, and the decision to thaw or not thaw is based on multiple factors, one being length of time to definitive treatment. Rewarming should not occur until there is guarantee of maintaining a warm environment. Refreezing must be avoided, because of the significant increase in tissue damage with each freeze-thaw cycle. Mobility is possible with a frozen extremity, and the goal is to mitigate the possibility of further trauma. If thawing is done, it should be done with a warm-water bath immersion avoiding the use of fire, space heaters, or other mechanical devices, because of the risk of thermal burn injuries. Additional field care includes pain control, administering ibuprofen, avoiding debridement of blisters, applying topical aloe vera if available, applying dry bulky dressings for protection, avoiding ambulation or use of affected extremity, and elevating the body part as able.[7,8,20]

Rewarming should be done in warm water heated and maintained between 37° and 40°C with an added mild antibacterial agent. This process may take 15 to 30 minutes and continues until tissues are flushed and pliable, signaling the end of vasoconstriction.[19,20,23,24]

Post-thaw care involving blisters remains controversial. Most recommend aspirating or debriding clear blisters, which indicate superficial injury, because of the prostaglandins and thromboxanes that may damage the underlying tissue. Hemorrhagic blisters represent structural damage to the dermal plexus and are generally left intact, as not doing so may lead to desiccation and presents an increased potential for infection.[19,20] The application of aloe vera, a potent antiprostaglandin agent, applied with dressing changes or every 6 hours, enhances tissue survival. Affected limbs should be loosely dressed and elevated to reduce edema. Edema is an indirect marker of endothelial integrity and plays a role in the pathogenesis of progressive dermal ischemia.[19,21] The cold-injured part is considered a tetanus-prone wound, and administering tetanus toxoid is indicated. The use of analgesics should be considered for pain management as necessary. Nonsteroidal anti-inflammatory drugs block the arachidonic pathway and decrease the production of prostaglandins and thromboxanes. Ibuprofen (12 mg/kg per day in divided doses) is recommended owing to its selective antiprostaglandin activity. Aspirin has been used, but may be less beneficial because it blocks all prostaglandins, including some prostacyclin that may promote wound healing. Systemic antibiotics are not routinely administered, although they should be given if signs and/or symptoms of infection occur. Fasciotomy may be indicated based on elevated compartment pressures (>37–40 mm Hg) and clinical judgment.[6–8,16,20,23,24]

Other interventions include performing daily hydrotherapy if needed for debridement, promoting active motion of the affected limb, providing a high-protein and high-calorie diet to encourage healing, recognizing and attending to psychosocial needs, and engaging a multidisciplinary team approach to improve long-term functional outcomes.[6,16,19,20]

There are anecdotal reports on the use of a hydrofiber silver dressing for frostbite patients. The hydrofiber dressing, used in thermal burns, forms a gel on contact with wound fluid to provide a moist wound-healing environment, manage exudates, help protect periwound skin, and reduce pain on removal of the dressing. The reported outcomes include decreased nursing time for dressing changes, decreased cost associated with multiple daily dressing changes, decreased pain with dressing changes, and improved patient satisfaction (D. Pomeroy RN, WOCN, oral communication, January 2012, Fairbanks Memorial Hospital).

Early surgical debridement is not recommended, because of the length of time it may take for demarcation of nonviable tissue. Tissue that initially appears nonviable may be restored through reperfusion once rewarming has been accomplished. Early surgical intervention has historically been thought to paradoxically injure recovering tissue and increase tissue loss. In the absence of gas gangrene, mummification occurs over 1 to 3 months, and the decision for definitive debridement versus allowing autoamputation can be made at this stage. Accepted indicators for early debridement include uncontrolled infection, gangrene, and clearly necrotic or nonfunctional tissue.[6,7,16,19]

The role of imaging has been to identify the need for and extent of debridement, and is a useful adjunct to clinical examination. Technetium-99 scintigraphy, magnetic resonance imaging, and magnetic resonance arteriography have been demonstrated in severe cases of frostbite to assist in more accurately defining the injury, and may be the most useful imaging modalities used in conjunction with the clinical presentation in determining the need and timing for surgery.[6–8,16,19,20]

Thrombolytic therapy is emerging as a treatment for severe frostbite injury that presents within 24 hours. The goal of therapy is to address microvascular thrombosis to salvage tissue at risk. Bruen and colleagues[27] demonstrated a reduction in digital amputation rates in patients receiving thrombolytic therapy, and calls it the first clinically significant advancement in the treatment of frostbite in more than 25 years. Only deep injuries with potential for significant morbidity should be considered for thrombolytic therapy because of potential for bleeding complications, compartment syndrome due to reperfusion associated edema, and failure to salvage tissue.[8,20] Thrombolytic therapy is ineffective in cold exposures for longer than 24 hours or in those cases with evidence of multiple freeze-thaw cycles.[7]

Other adjunctive therapies that have been examined include the use of low molecular weight dextran (LMWD) to decrease blood viscosity by preventing aggregation of red blood cells and mitigating the extent of tissue necrosis. Treatment using LMWD is beneficial if used in early treatment; however, it should not be used if the patient is being considered for thrombolytic therapy. The use of vasodilators to increase blood flow has been investigated, and a study from Europe showed a decrease in the rate of digit amputation with the use of iloprost, a synthetic prostacyclin that mimics the effects of a sympathectomy. Sympathectomy has been studied with limited and conflicting results and has not been shown to reduce tissue loss, but may have a role in the management of postfrostbite pain. Hyperbaric oxygen therapy has been successful with other types of wounds, but there are insufficient data to support recommendations for its use in the treatment of frostbite.[8,19,20]

LONG-TERM EFFECTS

Frostbite injury does not always lead to amputation, but can result in persistent symptoms that may last for years or even a lifetime. The long-term effects affect vasomotor function, nerve function, and/or the musculoskeletal system. The most commonly reported problem is chronic pain, probably as a result of vasomotor dysfunction. Cold hypersensitivity, paresthesias and sensory deficits, increased susceptibility to further cold injury, and hyperhidrosis in the affected parts are persistent problems. Other reported problems include muscle atrophy, premature closure of epiphyses in children causing growth stunting, decreased mineralization of bone, joint contractures, and

---

Box 1
Cold protection measures

Avoid environmental conditions with a risk of frostbite

Protect skin from exposure to wind and cold

Avoid sweating or getting extremities wet

Multilayer clothes for protection and insulation; avoid constriction

Use mittens to decrease hand heat loss

Use adjustable headgear for maximal coverage of exposed areas

Avoid substances (ie, alcohol, drugs) or conditions (hypoxia) that interfere with appropriate decision making regarding changing environmental conditions

Maintain peripheral warmth with use of chemical or electrical hand and foot warmers

Recognize frostnip and address it before it becomes more serious

Minimize duration of cold exposure

Maintain adequate nutrition and hydration

Avoid immobility

Avoid smoking

Be aware of personal risk factors (eg, medications, health issues, self-awareness)

Be prepared for the unexpected and/or accidental situations

Use appropriate measures for exposures to cold metal, gases, and so forth

Follow occupational cold risk management measures

Data from Refs.[1,6,20]

---

functional compromise secondary to amputations. Areas that have been frostbitten may have chronic ulceration issues and be prone to malignant squamous transformation.[6–8,16]

PREVENTION

Cold-weather environments present hazards resulting in higher risks of frostbite in comparison with other areas. Frostbite occurs when the local tissue perfusion is not capable of preventing freezing, because of tissue heat loss. Adequate perfusion and minimized heat loss are both required to prevent frostbite.[20] The primary cold-stress factors for outdoor activities are air temperature, wind speed, and wetness. Layering clothing, staying dry, and avoiding wind or protecting against it are essential actions in avoiding the risk of frostbite.[1,15]

There is a need to increase public awareness of the adverse effects of cold exposure. Assisting individuals in identifying contributing risk factors can lead to effective implementation of risk management and injury-prevention strategies. Populations that are at greatest risk for frostbite are children, elders, the homeless, and those with chronic diseases.[1] The measures for minimizing exposure of tissue to cold are listed in **Box 1**.

SUMMARY

Frostbite is an injury risk for those exposed to environmental extremes in cold-weather regions. Prevention is the first intervention, and providing risk-reduction education addressing the needs of vulnerable populations is essential. Greater understanding of the pathophysiology of frostbite has led to improved patient outcomes with treatment focused on rapid rewarming, aspiration or debridement of serous blisters, use of anti-inflammatory agents, and delayed surgical intervention. Thrombolytic therapy may contribute to improved outcomes in certain circumstances.

ACKNOWLEDGMENTS

The author extends thanks to Deb Pomeroy, who reviewed the article for clinical accuracy.

REFERENCES

1. Ikäheimo TM, Hassi J. Frostbites in circumpolar areas. Glob Health Action 2011;4:8456. http://dx.doi.org/10.3402/gha.v4i0.8456. Available at: http://www.globalhealthaction. net/index.php/gha/article/view/8456/12236. Accessed January 2, 2012.
2. Mills W, O'Malley J, Kappes B. Cold and freezing: a historical chronology of laboratory investigation and clinical experience. Alaska Med 1993;35:89–117.
3. Whayne T, DeBakey M. Cold injury: ground type. 1958. Available at: http://history. amedd.army.mil/booksdocs/wwii/ColdInjury/Chapter03.htm. Accessed January 30, 2012.
4. Rodway GW, McIntosh SE, Askew EW. Bradford Washburn's NEJM article "Frostbite: what it is-how to prevent it-emergency treatment"—historical background and commentary. Wilderness Environ Med 2011;22:177–81.
5. Hall A, Evans K, Pribyl S. Cold injury in the United States military population: current trends and comparison with past conflicts. J Surg Educ 2010;67:61–5.
6. Hallam MJ, Cubison T, Dheansa B, et al. Managing frostbite. BMJ 2010;341: 1151–6. http://dx.doi.org/10.1136/bmj.c5864.
7. Golant A, Nord RM, Paksima N, et al. Cold exposure injuries to the extremities. J Am Acad Orthop Surg 2008;16:704–15.
8. Grieve AW, Davis P, Dhillon S, et al. A clinical review of the management of frostbite. J R Army Med Corps 2011;157:73–8.
9. March P, Grose S. Frostbite: quick lesson. CINAHL Information Systems. 2011. Available at: http://web.ebscohost.com/ehost/pdfviewer/pdfviewer?vid=4&hid=11&sid=4657e591-66ac-4165-ba21-31cc976813dd%40sessionmgr14. Accessed January 20, 2012.
10. Emergency Nurses Association, Alaska chapter. Alaska Trauma Registry non-fatal trauma (2001–2005, 2004–2008, 2006–2010) documents. Available at: http://www.alaskaena.org/trauma.html. Accessed August 1, 2012.
11. Candler W, Ivey H. Cold weather injuries among U.S. soldiers in Alaska: a five year review. Mil Med 1997;162:788–91.
12. Erickson L, Rubertone M, Brundage J. Cold weather injuries, active duty soldiers. MSMR 2000;6:2–8. Available at: http://afhsc.army.mil/msmr. Accessed February 6, 2012.
13. Armed Forces Health Surveillance Center. Cold injuries, active component members, U.S. Armed Forces, July 2000-June 2005. MSMR 2005;11:7–11. Available at: http://afhsc.army.mil/msmr. Accessed February 6, 2012.
14. Armed Forces Health Surveillance Center. Update: cold weather injuries, U.S. Armed Forces, July 2006-June 2011. MSMR 2011;18:14–8. Available at: http://afhsc.army.mil/msmr. Accessed February 6, 2012.
15. Castellini J, Young A, Ducharme M, et al. Prevention of cold injuries during exercise. Med Sci Sports Exerc 2006;38:2012–29.

16. Bjerke H, Tevar A. Frostbite. 2012. Available at: http://emedicine.medscape.com/article/194957-overview. Accessed January 12, 2012.
17. Mohr W, Jenabzadeh K, Ahrenholz D. Cold injury. Hand Clin 2009;25:481–96.
18. National Weather Service. Wind chill chart. Available at: http://www.nws.noaa.gov/om/windchill/index.shtml. Accessed January 2, 2012.
19. Murphy J, Banwell P, Roberts A, et al. Frostbite: pathogenesis and treatment. J Trauma 2000;48:171–8.
20. McIntosh S, Hamonko M, Freer L, et al. Wilderness Medical Society practice guidelines for the prevention and treatment of frostbite. Wilderness Environ Med 2011;22:156–66.
21. Goertz O, Hirsch T, Buschhaus B, et al. Intravital pathophysiologic comparison of frostbite and burn injury in a murine model. J Surg Res 2011;167:e395–401. http://dx.doi.org/10.106/j.jss.2011.01.034.
22. Mills W, Whaley R. Frostbite: experience with rapid rewarming and ultrasonic therapy, Part 1. 1960. Alaska Med 1993;35:6–9.
23. Mills W. Frostbite: a discussion of the problem and a review of an Alaskan experience. Alaska Med 1993;35:29–49.
24. Zafren K. Revised cold injury & cold water near drowning guidelines. 2012. Available at: www.hss.state.ak.us/dph/emergency/ems/Assets/Downloads/cold_inj.ppt. Accessed February 19, 2012.
25. Cauchy E, Chetaille E, Marchand V, et al. Retrospective study of 70 cases of severe frostbite lesions: a proposed new classification scheme. Wilderness Environ Med 2001;12:248–55.
26. Paton B. A history of frostbite treatment. Int J Circumpolar Health 2000;59:99–107.
27. Bruen K, Ballard J, Morris S, et al. Reduction of the incidence of amputation in frostbite injury with thrombolytic therapy. Arch Surg 2007;142:546–53.

Rural Trauma Challenges in Alaska

Christie E. Artuso, EdD, RN, CNRN

KEYWORDS

- Winter trauma • Snowboarding trauma • Snowmobile trauma • Rural trauma
- Arctic trauma

KEY POINTS

- Rural trauma in Alaska during the winter months requires a coordinated highly skilled approach for rescue, recovery, resuscitation, and transport to tertiary care centers. Injuries vary by sport and trauma.
- Early assessment and resuscitation rely on minimizing delays.
- Prehospital care is initiated by first responder and rescue teams, with advanced medical care by critical care transport teams.

SIGNIFICANCE OF TRAUMA IN ALASKA

Traumatic injury is the fifth leading cause of death in the United States and the leading cause of death and disability among individuals age 1 to 44.[1] Traumatic injury results in more than $400 billion each year in medical costs and lost productivity with more than 29 million individuals treated each year in emergency departments.[2] Improving outcomes for trauma victims in rural settings presents unique challenges to health care providers and health care systems throughout the United States. Alaska adds 586,412 square miles, rapidly changing weather conditions, geographic barriers, and extreme sports to the routine difficulties faced by other rural communities, creating a setting that promises an unprecedented platform for emergency rescue, transport, and resuscitation. In 2011, the US Census Bureau estimated the population of Alaska at 722,718 with approximately 40% of the population residing in Anchorage, the state's largest city.[3] The 3 largest hospitals are located in Anchorage and most serious trauma would be transported to one of these medical centers. There are 31 health care facilities throughout the state, including 11 community hospitals, 13 critical access hospitals, and 7 specialty or military facilities. More than 25% of Alaskans live in communities of fewer than 1000 people. Seventy-five percent of Alaskan communities are unconnected by a road to a hospital. Health care systems are faced with

The author has nothing to disclose.
Neuroscience Services, Providence Alaska Medical Center, 3200 Providence Drive, AK 99519, USA
E-mail address: Christie.artuso@providence.org

the challenges of meeting the needs of the dispersed population of this vast rural state while overcoming geographic barriers, providing service across mountain ranges, volcanoes, and encountering extreme weather conditions, as well as communication challenges owing to lack of cell and radio coverage.

Patient outcomes are directly related to the time elapsed between traumatic injury and properly delivered definitive care. Although fewer motor vehicle accidents occur in rural areas, more than two-thirds of the deaths related to motor vehicle trauma occur on rural roads.[4] Improved mortality and morbidity is related to rapid field assessment and immediate transport to an appropriate health care facility.[5] A coordinated model for assessment and triage to an appropriate facility is an essential component for the achievement of optimal patient outcomes.[6] The vast wilderness, geography, weather, and limited health care facilities in Alaska present unprecedented challenges for emergency responders and the health care system. Local response to rural trauma in Alaska is coordinated through a knowledgeable dispatch system often using specialized and highly trained rescue teams in addition to advanced life support personnel who may travel to the site of the trauma by helicopter, fixed wing airplane, or Lear jet. The ability to place qualified health care providers at the scene can be inhibited by visibility, unsettled weather patterns, geography, and available, appropriate runways requiring additional equipment and traversing difficult terrain. If aircraft are unable to land close to the scene, transport time will be increased, affecting the patient's outcome.[7] The medical crew travels with survival packs, including cold weather gear and arctic outerwear, ready-to-eat meals (commonly referred to as MREs) emergency medical equipment, snow shoes for post-holing, and crampons for the icy conditions found on glaciers and in the mountainous areas of Alaska. Highly trained rescue teams often facilitate reaching the victim or victims and provide additional support, safety, and security for the medical team.

RANGE OF INJURY

Rural trauma in Alaska ranges from minor musculoskeletal injuries associated with hiking, snow-shoeing, snow-boarding and skiing to severe hypothermia and asphyxiation often seen in victims of avalanches. Motor vehicle accidents also include injuries sustained in snow machine and all-terrain vehicle accidents. Alcohol is a common denominator in many of these accidents during the long dark winter months in Alaska, complicating the resuscitative efforts and mortality rates. The patient's access to appropriate care, the time that it takes to rescue a victim from the scene of an accident or trauma, and the circumstances surrounding transport to tertiary care may impact the patient's outcome more significantly than that initial injury itself.

SKIING AND SNOWBOARDING

Alpine skiing, cross-country skiing, and snowboarding are popular winter activities throughout Alaska. Although there are only a few designated ski resorts with chair lifts and ski patrol staff, many individuals enjoy the sports in unchartered terrain and on ungroomed trails. Experience and the level of the individual's ability are often correlated with the risk for injury.[8] The most common type of traumatic injury associated with alpine skiing, snowboarding, and cross-country skiing is extremity trauma. The physical forces that produce injury in this population include acceleration/deceleration (the body making contact with another object while both are in motion), shearing, tearing, distraction, rotation, flexion, compression, and penetration. Skiers are more likely to suffer lower-extremity trauma and snowboarders are more likely to sustain upper-extremity trauma.[9] High-speed impacts with another individual or a stationary object can cause serious closed or open fractures of the femur, tibia, fibula, and patella. Skiers and snowboarders also risk head, spine, and torso trauma from collisions or impact with unexpected changes in the terrain.[10] These injuries may include vertebral fractures or blunt trauma to the kidney, resulting in internal bleeding. Penetrating trauma is also seen from ski poles, tree branches, or other sharp objects that may enter the body at a high rate of speed.

SAFETY AT THE SCENE

In every trauma situation, the safety of the scene is the first priority.[9] First responders will assess the scene and determine potential risk for rescuers and the members of the medical team. In Alaska, the first responders may be family and friends with little or no emergency training, community members, volunteer emergency medical staff, or local law enforcement personnel. Paramedics or registered nurses with critical care, emergency, and/or flight certifications will respond to the scene after notification by first responders; however, the distance between communities may result in a significant delay in medical response. It is not uncommon in these distant and rural settings for the central dispatch team to call a military rescue squad or a National Guard search-and-rescue team to assist in access to victims at the scene. Common issues at the scene may be steep terrain, waist-deep snow requiring snow shoes and aerial support, ice, and crevices. Many of the back-country scenes are accessible only by air or snow machine, requiring collaborative and coordinated efforts for successful rescue and resuscitation. After the scene is secure and first responders reach the victim or victims, priority assessment includes presence of an airway, breathing, and any circulatory issues, including fractures resulting in volume loss or the potential for internal injuries. Depending on the safety at the scene, first responders and emergency medical service rescue team members may evacuate the victim using necessary equipment, including immobilization devices and sleds, allowing for relocation to a safer environment. Other issues include the distance to the nearest landing strip or unrestricted area for helicopter landing, and mechanisms that can be used to transport the victim from the scene to the location where an aircraft waits to transport to 1 of the 2 tertiary care facilities in Anchorage.

PRIMARY ASSESSMENT

The field evaluation includes assessment of disability by establishing a baseline mental status and level of consciousness. Extreme temperatures also pose the risk for hypothermia, which may affect the patient's mental status and level of consciousness. Hypothermia occurs when the core body temperature falls below 95°F. More than two-thirds of all trauma victims are hypothermic at hospital arrival regardless of weather conditions. When the body has sustained severe traumatic injury, the metabolic rate decreases, resulting in a decrease in tissue perfusion and oxygenation. Core body temperature decreases as the body fails to produce enough heat, leading to hypothermia.[11] Alcohol also reduces the patient's ability to react appropriately to conditions and may increase the risk for the development of hypothermia.[12]

During assessment and transport, medical personnel recognize the risk for frostbite often associated with hypothermia and exposure to the cold. Although most patients may have been dressed appropriately for their activity, removal of clothing to assess an injury contributes to exposure and subsequent risk for frostbite. Wet clothing is a poor insulator and may lead to frostbite. Early interventions include removal of wet clothing, minimizing additional heat loss, and protection from further exposure. Rewarming is often delayed until the therapy can be coordinated at a tertiary care center. Alcohol consumption may also contribute to the early development of frostbite in trauma victims in the arctic environment.

TRANSPORT AND ASSESSMENT

As clinicians monitor the patient's status during transport, changes in mental status are evaluated for significance related to a deteriorating neurologic status related to head injury or a secondary change in mental status related to hypothermia. External body temperatures are often decreased and core body temperatures difficult to assess during transport and flight. Keeping the patient warm is a priority; however, this priority may impede easy access to injured parts and visual assessment. A coordinated approach is used to maintain normothermia and ongoing assessment for change in physical condition related to injury. Thermal blankets, body heat, and a heated cabin during transport are all used to prevent further hypothermia. A secondary assessment may be performed after the immobilized patient is safely secure and in transport; however, the priority is often focused on time and rapid transport to the tertiary care facility.

Patients with volume depletion secondary to blood loss from serious injuries will require fluid resuscitation; however, traditional intravenous fluid resuscitation may be challenging. Temperatures fluctuate and fall as low as 40 to 60°F below zero. Crystalloid and colloid fluids will freeze after only a few seconds of exposure to these extreme temperatures. The priorities for emergency care often deviate from the traditional assessment, primary and secondary surveys, and resuscitative efforts to immobilization and evacuation from the scene with interventions and resuscitation based on conditions. Intravenous fluid bags and tubing must be shielded from exposure in these extreme conditions to prevent ice crystal formation and subsequent loss of intravenous access.[13]

MOTOR VEHICLE ACCIDENTS: SNOW MACHINES

Motor vehicle accidents are another source of trauma in Alaska; however, many of these accidents are related to snowmobiles, commonly referred to as snow machines in Alaska, all-terrain vehicles, and off-road trucks. Most snow machine accidents are caused by natural obstacles, excessive speed, and alcohol intoxication.[14] Snow machine use is minimally regulated, with no laws regarding operator training, helmets, or set speed limits.[15] A study evaluating snowmobile injuries in the northwest found that most patients were treated in the emergency department and did not require hospitalization. Some, however, can be fatal. Injuries can include both orthopedic and nonorthopedic injuries. Common nonorthopedic injuries include open wounds to the head, back strains, and various contusions of the lower extremities and trunk. Emergency care at the scene includes assessment for hemorrhage and volume loss, and stabilization and immobilization of the injured extremity. Additional interventions are determined based on the estimated transport time, the distance from the site of the trauma to the tertiary care facility, and the overall clinical condition of the patient. Hypothermia is also a concern, as snow machine incidents often involve submersion and exposure to frigid waters.

Dispatch calls related to snow machine accidents are challenging and unpredictable. The dispatch notification call may simply refer to the need for medical care with minimal information about the victim and even the location. One call came on a midwinter day requesting medical assistance for a victim of a snow machine accident with cardiopulmonary resuscitation in progress. The specific location of the accident and victim was unknown; however, the group had been riding in a popular rural area located between mountains in a large mountain range spanning 300 acres. Although State Troopers in Alaska use snow machines, at the time of dispatch, the state troopers had been unsuccessful in locating the party or the victim. The group did not have a Global Positioning System (GPS) device or satellite phone and cellular service was intermittent. The Bell 212 Twin Huey Helicopter was dispatched depending on a relay of information between central dispatch and the state troopers searching for the group. After circling the area for 20 minutes, the pilot located the group huddled around a fire; however, was unable to locate the victim. After landing, the medical team donned their snow shoes and post-holed toward the group. Upon arrival, they were told that the victim was approximately 50 feet away from the fire.

The primary survey revealed a pulseless cold victim with no obvious sign of outward injury. When asked why they had stopped their resuscitative efforts, the group stated that their efforts seemed hopeless. Two snow machines had been jumping and crossing paths when the ski of one snow machine clipped the helmet of the victim, ejecting him from his machine. The medical team pronounced the patient deceased at the scene. When turning the victim to assess for further injury, it was obvious that a head injury and high-level spine injury had likely caused an immediate death. Blood loss was contained beneath the victim from a head wound at the base of the skull. Despite the rapid response and highly skilled team, clinical outcomes are not always positive.

Avalanches are also associated with snow machine injuries and winter trauma in rural settings. An avalanche occurs when the weight of the snow increases and slides from the slope of a mountain. Variations in weather, temperature, slope steepness, slope orientation (north or south), wind, vegetation, and snow pack conditions affect the likelihood of an avalanche.[16] Victims of an avalanche often sustain orthopedic injuries and asphyxiation from the weight of the snow. Rescue efforts are focused toward locating the victim and providing access to oxygen as quickly as possible. The use of a bag-valve-mask device is also challenging in the arctic environment when temperatures exceed 30° to 40°F below zero. The mechanisms inside these ventilator devices may freeze, affecting the rescuer's ability to provide ventilation. In these situations, the priority shifts from airway and breathing to rapid transport from one location to another, where exposure to these extreme temperatures is minimized and the environment conducive to ventilator support. From 2001 through 2010, there were 37 avalanche-related deaths in Alaska.[17] Avalanche beacons are often worn by winter sports enthusiasts; however, the depth of snow following an avalanche may impede a rapid recovery and subsequent resuscitation.

On-road motor vehicle accidents also contribute to rural trauma and often result in multiple injury scenarios, including orthopedic injuries, penetrating and blunt trauma, and traumatic brain injury. Response to a motor vehicle accident follows the same guidelines in rural settings, with safety at the scene achieved before resuscitative efforts. In rural communities, communication is also an issue, with limited cellular service affecting connectivity with additional resources. Satellite technology facilitates rescue and emergency crew communication with their medic base and their dispatch teams.

Winter travel, snow, and circumstances surrounding motor vehicle accidents and off-road accidents often affect the severity of the injuries, the outcome, and the response. Multiple victims may be involved in a single accident, requiring triage at the scene and critical decision making for transport. A case that illustrates this point involved 3 victims and a roll-over vehicle in a rural area: 1 victim with a possible head injury, 1 with a knee injury, and 1 with a possible spine injury. It was a clear, sunny day in March; however, the snow was several feet deep. Lift-off time was never greater than 10 minutes with travel to this geographic area of 60 minutes. The helicopter landed in a clearing and the flight nurse scanned the area for the actual location of the accident. The vehicle and victims were at the bottom of a 25-foot snow-covered embankment. While the pilot and paramedic selected a longer but safer route to transport the stretcher and equipment bags, the flight nurse post-holed down the embankment toward the first victim. The area contained strong fumes and a tarp covered an apparent gas spill. The 28-year-old female victim was awake, lying on her back with her feet and legs bent at a 180° angle awkwardly positioned at the right side of her face. Her head was turned toward the left side of her body and her left arm was draped in the opposite direction, over her face toward her right. She was breathing. When the bystanders were questioned, they stated that they had attempted to move the arm from its awkward position; however, the patient had become apneic. The patient had no sensation or movement in 4 extremities and serious cervical injury was suspected. Oxygen was administered through a simple mask while the pilot, paramedic, and flight nurse stabilized the cervical region and boarded the patient on the stretcher. As they moved the patient, a thick piece of hair lifted, exposing three-quarters of a pearly white skull. Despite the injuries, there was no outward sign of bleeding. The patient denied pain. As the pilot and paramedic began to move the immobilized victim toward the helicopter, the flight nurse assessed the remaining 2 victims. Both were stable with minor injuries and the decision was made to send ground transport crews for medical care. The time on the ground was 15 minutes from landing to liftoff.

Shortly after liftoff, the patient developed a pulse of 50 and a blood pressure of 90/42. These clinical manifestations were consistent with neurogenic shock, a distributive form of progressive shock related to the disruption of autonomic pathways resulting from high spinal cord injury. Immediate interventions included warmed fluid boluses to improve intravascular volume and raise the core body temperature. Despite numerous attempts, communication with the emergency department base was sporadic and ineffective. It is not uncommon for a flight team to experience difficulties related to direct communication with physicians in the emergency department. Upon arrival, the trauma team at the tertiary care facility stabilized the patient and transferred her to a Level I Trauma Center 1500 miles south of Anchorage for advanced neurosurgical care and rehabilitation. The patient survived without additional complication; however, remains a quadriplegic.

TRAUMATIC BRAIN INJURY

In many instances, the evaluation of a trauma patient's scope of injury will include the assumption that a traumatic brain injury will be a component of the overall assessment. Even without a loss of consciousness, the nature of injury accompanying skiing, snowboarding, and winter sports–related traumas will result in subsequent minor or moderate head injury. Although the statewide average for traumatic brain injury is similar to the national average in the United States, the incidence in rural Alaska is 4 times the national average.[18] Clinical evaluation at the scene may not provide definitive information; however, a detailed history, the mechanism of injury, a physical examination, and most, importantly, clinical judgment will facilitate an accurate clinical diagnosis.[19] Traumatic brain injury may be present with or without the use of protective gear, including helmets. Victims may have sustained a linear or depressed skull fracture, which may or may not be evident at the scene of the incident. First responders and the medical team perform a thorough physical examination and neurologic assessment as a baseline, with periodic reassessment of the Glasgow Coma Scale and ongoing assessment of the airway, breathing patterns, and oxygenation.[20] Ongoing assessment during extended air transport presents challenges for clinicians, affecting the reliability of data, difficulty assessing subtle changes in condition, and the risk for increased intracranial pressure related to altitude.[21]

Medical crews responding to rural trauma in Alaska are usually composed of a pilot, flight nurse, and a paramedic or a pilot and 2 flight nurses. In some states, a physician may be a member of the crew. Critical-care air-transport teams bring a higher level of practice to the scene of a traumatic injury, including chest decompression by needle or tube thoracostomy, rapid sequence intubation, central lines, portable point-of-care laboratory testing, and pericardiocentesis. These procedures are often not available in rural hospital or local clinic settings, but provide valuable information that facilitates accurate clinical decisions before arrival at the tertiary care facility. Air transport and emergency rescue in wilderness regions serves to decrease mortality by supporting a higher level of clinical care and intervention for trauma victims.[22]

Winter trauma in Alaska encompasses diverse clinical scenarios varying in severity and outcome. Many victims are young, with injuries related to winter sports and activities including alpine skiing, hiking, cross-country skiing, snowboarding, and snow machining. Avalanches pose an additional threat and may cause injury to individuals who are walking, hiking, driving or enjoying any of the popular sports. Other less common sources of injury include ice skating, outdoor hockey, and ice fishing, with subsequent trauma related to exposure and hypothermia. Prehospital care is often initiated by first responders and highly skilled rescue teams, with subsequent advanced medical care by a highly trained critical-care transport team. Outcomes are affected by distances between locations and the few tertiary care facilities in the state, variable weather conditions, extreme temperatures, limited runways and landing sites, and delays from complicated rescues and extrications. Despite these barriers, access to tertiary care is the result of highly sophisticated coordinated emergency services and collaborative efforts between private and government agencies.

ACKNOWLEDGMENTS

A special thank you to Ella Goss, RN, for sharing her insights and experiences from her years as a front-line flight nurse in Alaska.

REFERENCES

1. Prevention CF. Fast stats. In Centers for Disease Control and Prevention. Available at: www.cdc.gov/nchs/fastats/acc-inj.htm. Accessed February 5, 2012.
2. Prevention CF. Injury prevention, control. In Centers for Disease Control and Prevention. Available at: http://www.cdc.gov/injury/overview/leading_cod.html. Accessed February 5, 2012.
3. US Census Bureau. State and county quick facts. In U.S. Census Bureau. Available at: http://quickfacts.census.gov/qfd/states/02000.html. Accessed January 28, 2012.
4. Rawlinson C, Crews P. Access to quality health services in rural areas—emergency medical services: a literature review. Washington, DC: Healthy People; 2010.
5. American College of Surgeons. Resources for optimal care of the injured patient. Chicago: American College of Surgeons; 2006.
6. Hankins DG. Air medical transport of trauma patients. Prehosp Emerg Care 2006; 10:324–7.

7. Nakstad AR, Strand T, Sandberg M. Landing sites and intubation may influence helicopter emergency medical services on-scene time. J Emerg Med 2011;40: 651–7.

8. Langran MS. Increased injury risk among first-day skiers, snowboarders, and ski-boarders. Am J Sports Med 2004;32:96–103.

9. Laskowski-Jones L, Jones L. Winter emergencies: managing ski and snowboard injuries. Nursing 2009;42(8):25–30.

10. Calle SC, Evans JT. Snowboarding trauma. J Pediatr Surg 1995;30:791–4.

11. Langran M, Selvaraj S. Increased injury risk among first-day skiers, snow-boarders, and ski-boarders. Am J Sports Med 2004;32:96–103.

12. Accidental hypothermia. Emerg Med Reports. Atlanta (GA): AHC Media, LLC; 2009.

13. Laskowski-Jones L. Responding to winter emergencies. Nursing 2000;30:4–40.

14. The Alaska Bureau of Vital Statistics. Unintentional Injury Deaths for Alaska. In the Alaska Bureau of Vital Statistics. Available at: http://www.hss.state.ak.us/dph/bvs/death_statistics/Unintentional_Injury_Census/body.html. Accessed October 27, 2011.

15. American Council of Snowmobile Associations. State Laws and Rules. In American Council of Snowmobile Associations (2012). Available at: http://www.snowmobilers.org/facts_statelaws.html. Accessed February 6, 2012.

16. Alaska Department of Natural Resources. Avalanches. In Alaska Department of Natural Resources: Division of Parks, Outdoor Recreation. 2012. Available at: http://dnr.alaska.gov/parks/safety/avalanch.htm. Accessed February 10, 2012.

17. Colorado Avalanche Information Center. Avalanche accident statistics. In Colorado Avalanche Information Center. Available at: http://avalanche.state.co.us/acc/acc_images/Slide7.JPG. Accessed February 12, 2012.

18. Alaska Brain Injury Network. In traumatic brain injury Alaska data. Available at: http://www.alaskabraininjury.org/index.cfm?fa=documents_overview&doctype=35. Accessed March 22, 2012.

19. Easter JS, Grossman SA, Woodruff MM, et al. When the rules do not work: head injury without loss of consciousness. J Emerg Med 2008;35:77–80.

20. Barker E. Neuroscience nursing: a spectrum of care. 3rd edition. St Louis (MO): Mosby; 2008.

21. Singh JM, MacDonald RD, Bronskill SE, et al. Incidence and predictors of critical events during urgent air-medical transport. CMAJ 2009;181:579–84.

22. Kaufmann M, Moser B, Lederer W. Changes in injury patterns and severity in a helicopter air-rescue system over a 6-year period. Wilderness Environ Med 2006;17:8–14.

Journey of a Survivor of Near Drowning, Polymicrobial Pneumonia, and Acute Respiratory Distress Syndrome

Margaret M. Ecklund, MS, RN, CCRN, ACNP-BC[a],*, Gary Wahl, MD[b],
Alexandra V. Yamshchikov, MD[c], Michael S. Smith[a]

KEYWORDS

- Near drowning • Pneumonia • ARDS • Progressive mobility

KEY POINTS

- Near drowning can result in a polymicrobial pneumonia with unpredictable disease course.
- Acute lung injury requires ventilation support based on lung compliance and response to pressure delivery to support oxygenation.
- Bronchopleural fistulas may develop as a consequence of cavitary lesions from fungal infiltrates and are exacerbated by the pressure of mechanical ventilation.
- Progressive mobility limits functional deconditioning and has a positive effect on full recovery to baseline.
- Social networking provides an outlet for families for coping and can be a tool for recovery.

THE EVENT

Barb felt good on the morning of December 3. The temperature was $-2°C$ and it was cloudy, with no precipitation. She was walking in a local park with her 2 golden retrievers. Twenty minutes into the walk, she began to feel dizzy and called her husband, Mike, on her cell phone. Within 10 to 15 minutes, he arrived at the park at the spot she had identified, and immediately saw Barb lying motionless. She was clearly visible wearing a bright red coat. When he got out of the car and ran to her,

The authors have nothing to disclose.
[a] Pulmonary Care, Rochester General Health System, 1425 Portland Avenue, Rochester, NY 14621, USA; [b] Department of Pulmonary Medicine, Rochester General Health System, Rochester General Hospital, 1425 Portland Avenue, Rochester, NY 14621, USA; [c] Infectious Diseases Unit, Rochester General Hospital, University of Rochester School of Medicine, 1425 Portland Avenue, Rochester, NY 14621, USA
* Corresponding author.
E-mail address: margaret.ecklund@rochestergeneral.org

he could see that she was face down in about 15 cm of water. There was heavy precipitation the night before and standing water was everywhere. He turned her over to find her gray and unresponsive. She was not breathing.

He began artificial respiration and the first breath in caused her to regurgitate water. With each subsequent breath, he heard breathing, but quickly realized it was only his own breath escaping her lungs through her teeth, causing a buzzing sound. His cell phone fell into the puddle and did not function. He was unable to summon help in the deserted winter park. He began to scream loudly for help as he provided her breaths. A driver in a car on the main highway eventually heard his cries and came over to call the emergency medical system (EMS). At about the time that the other driver arrived, Barb began to breathe on her own and her skin turned pink.

The EMS arrived and found her to have shallow, spontaneous breathing, a pulse of 72 beats per minute (bpm), and a blood pressure (BP) of 127/63 mm Hg. She was supported with 100% oxygen for transport to the hospital. As she was being cared for, Mike gathered the dogs and noted pain in his right leg. He also required assessment and treatment in the same emergency room, and was eventually diagnosed with a complete quadriceps tear. This injury required surgical repair, follow-up treatment of infection, and prolonged therapy.

INTENSIVE CARE UNIT COURSE

Barb was intubated and supported with mechanical ventilation. Her temperature on arrival to the emergency room was 32.6°C. Her lactic acid level was 9.8 mmol/L (0.4–2.0 mmol/L) on admission. Placed in a warming device, she was transported to the intensive care unit (ICU). She was minimally responsive for the first 7 days. The initial chest computed tomography (CT) scan showed patchy bilateral airspace opacities consistent with pneumonia or pulmonary hemorrhage. Intravenous trimethoprim/ sulfamethoxazole was started. Nutrition was administered via a small-bore feeding tube and calculated to her needs based on weight. Enoxaprin subcutaneous provided deep vein thrombosis (DVT) prevention. Ventilator-associated pneumonia (VAP) bundle prevention included elevation of the head of the bed with routine oral care. Pantoprazole provided stress ulcer prevention. VAP prevention was instituted and early progressive mobility was achieved with bed to chair positioning and minimized sedation. Multidisciplinary planning helped achieve the goals of care.

By day 10, she was showing stability and improved interaction. She was extubated and supported with oxygen. Her left eye was cloudy, and keratitis was discovered secondary to a contact lens that had not been removed after the collapse. Her right lens likely fell out in the puddle. The ophthalmology team recommendations included ophthalmic care including antibiotic and steroid drops with lubricating ointment.

At day 11, her hypoxia required treatment with supplemental oxygen, which progressed to the need for reintubation. Respiratory therapist combined with nurses to promote optimal oxygen delivery and positioning for airway clearance. The course was complicated with critical hypoxia, ventilation difficulty, leukocytosis, and fever. A chest CT scan showed a small cavitary lesion in the left upper lobe with nodular opacities. *Legionella* was the suspected organism causing the pneumonia. However, concern arose that water aspirated during the near-drowning experience was likely contaminated by soil and excrement of horses and dogs. With this setback, vancomycin, amphotericin, and imipenem were initiated for polymicrobial coverage.

Despite prophylaxis with low-molecular-weight heparin, she developed a right leg DVT, therefore intravenous anticoagulation and oral warfarin therapies were started. A retrievable inferior vena cava (IVC) filter was placed by interventional radiology.

Supraventricular tachycardia (SVT) developed on day 15. With a heart rate of 200 bpm and systolic BP of 90 mm Hg, administration of adenosine brought the heart rate to 120 bpm. Adenosine was used for initial treatment to unmask the underlying rhythm, followed by metroprolol, which controlled heart rate, revealing an underlying sinus tachycardia.

During week 3, increased peak airway pressures and persistent hypoxia led to the diagnosis of adult respiratory distress syndrome (ARDS). Airway pressure release ventilation (APRV) was implemented over the following days with marginal improvement in oxygenation despite the delivery of high fraction of inspired oxygen and significant airway pressures. On day 21, the mode was changed to pressure control ventilation (PCV) with continued high oxygen needs, and moderate pressures to support volume delivery. Volumes varied with the attempt to support oxygen and prevent barotrauma, (trauma to the lung). The changes were based on respiratory therapist and physician collaboration.

A tracheostomy was considered after 21 days of intubation for ongoing airway access. The first operating room attempt was challenged by severe hypoxia. The procedure was aborted and she was returned to the ICU with full ventilation. A second surgical attempt for the tracheostomy tube was successful 48 h later. A size 7 French single cannula air cuffed tube was placed successfully.

Ventilation and oxygenation seemed to improve after tracheostomy and she seemed more comfortable. However, on day 23, Barb developed sudden-onset dyspnea with absent right-sided breath sounds. A chest radiograph revealed a large right pneumothorax. A large-bore chest tube was placed at the bedside with resultant lung reexpansion. At day 24 of the hospitalization, severe hypoxia prompted a chest CT scan. The CT findings of multiple cavity lesions and right pneumothorax despite the chest tube caused concern for a bronchopleural fistula. The CT scan was very different from earlier scans. A filling defect in the right upper lobe cystic lesion was consistent with an aspergilloma, and a diagnosis of *Aspergillus fumigatus* was made. This development led to another chest tube being placed, with symptom resolution. Antiinfectives changed from imipenem to levaquin. Amphotericin was changed to caspofungin, followed by voriconazole because of the resistant mold.

By day 27, her improvement was dramatic and weaning became more successful. At this point, sedation was changed to oral benzodiazepines and she was able to mobilize to the chair. Nurses coordinated with respiratory therapists to allow her to move safely with the airway and ventilator tubing. Continuous positive airway pressure (CPAP) with pressure support of 5 cm and oxygen delivery of 0.5 were required for respiratory support from day 27 to day 33. She progressed to being clinically ready to move from the ICU to the step-down unit.

PULMONARY STEP-DOWN UNIT CHALLENGES

The remaining 2 months of Barb's hospital course were on the pulmonary step-down unit. During this time, as she weaned from mechanical ventilation, the tracheostomy was removed, and her mobility increased and progressed to oral nutrition. However, more challenges of recurrent pneumothorax, further infections, recurrent SVT, and malnutrition complicated her course.

Spontaneous breathing trials were successful, with the support of high-flow oxygen delivery with humidification to the tracheostomy tube. The tracheostomy tube was changed to a smaller size 6 French tight to shaft silicone tube that allowed intermittent use of a speaking valve with cuff deflation. Clearing secretions was not an issue for Barb, and she maintained adequate oxygenation on levels of 0.6 to 0.7 inspired fraction of oxygen delivery, from day 33 to 40. Improving strength and mobility with a strong cough allowed for periods of tracheostomy tube plugging, which was accomplished by placing an occlusive cap over the tube with airflow around the perimeter of the tube while deflating the cuff. Her oxygen needs diminished to 4 to 6 L per minute by nasal cannula. From days 40 to 47 of hospital stay, she showed adequate oxygenation and successful secretion clearance. The tracheostomy tube was removed and stoma allowed closure by granulation.

She developed a urinary tract infection, despite no recent catheterization. The organism isolated was a vancomycin-resistant enterococcus, and was treated with oral linezolid. Contact isolation added a step to care and emotional isolation for her, which the health care team responded to by supporting her feelings. She continued with voriconazole for the identified pulmonary organism, Scedosporium. Piperacillin/tazobactam was added to cover Pseudomonas isolated in her sputum, clinically evident with fevers and leukocytosis. The piperacillin /tazobactam was later changed to oral ciprofloxacin.

Heart rate monitoring and BP surveillance were important during the period of progressive mobility, at the 1-month to 3-month points of her recovery. Because her resting heart rate was 100 to 120 bpm, increases in the rate of 10 to 20 bpm caused concern for decreased cardiac output and hemodynamic instability. Ongoing treatment of tachycardia for Barb was achieved with oral metroprolol. BP ranges of 90/50 to 98/50 mm Hg produced no symptomatic effects of hypotension.

For Barb, the initial few weeks after the pneumothorax were tenuous. Oxygenation was marginal as she spontaneously breathed off ventilator support. Any activity would cause tachycardia, high work of breathing, and oxygen desaturation. Any impendence of the chest tube patency would precipitate an oxygen decrease and distress. The multidisciplinary team of respiratory therapists, nurses, and physical therapists organized the room to allow movement within the room without obstruction of the chest tube water seal system: a challenge with limited floor space! Bright orange tubing labels and flow-meter alerts helped to identify the multiple clear tubes within the room. Another 2 weeks (day 41) passed with limited pulmonary healing, therefore a third chest tube was inserted as the second one was removed, resulting in full right lung expansion. With improved nutrition, the bronchopleural fistula healed and the chest tubes were pulled at week 9 (day 69) of the hospital stay. Pain control at chest tube sites was managed with oral narcotics. Free of the chest tube, she was walking longer distances and supplemental oxygen and rehabilitation options outside of the hospital were being considered.

Throughout the ICU and early step-down course, Barb's nutritional needs were met using a small-bore feeding tube, with enteral feedings calculated by the clinical dietitian for her needs. She had adequate tolerance but had suboptimal protein levels, so additional protein supplements were provided. When she passed her oral swallowing evaluation, she began an oral diet, but transitioned with nighttime feedings to meet her high requirements. During the final month of stay, she had her entire intake by the oral route, with careful menu selection and protein supplementation.

Barb developed a fever, leukocytosis, and watery diarrhea on day 74. Her stool was positive for Clostridium difficile toxin and oral vancomycin was implemented for a 2-week course. Gut recolonization was initiated with yogurt, to restore normal gastrointestinal flora.

During the night of hospital day 81, she awoke with a heavy chest feeling, describing it as: "An elephant on my chest." Supraventricular tachycardia was the rhythm with a rate of 180 bpm, and BP of 88/49 mm Hg. Adenosine converted the rhythm back to sinus tachycardia with a rate of 110 bpm. She suffered no ill effects. A cardiology evaluation led to a work-up including an electrophysiology study (EP) with ablation of the accessory pathway. She tolerated the procedure well. The team's hope was that the SVT caused the initial collapse in the park, and that cause was diagnosed and treated.

Lubrication of the eye, erythromycin, and steroid eye drops were part of the treatment plan for ongoing keratitis continued over the course of her hospital stay. Barb's vision was affected because of the keratitis and her outdated eyeglasses prescription. As the eye healed, the eyeglasses were not correcting her vision and caused frustration. A close friend provide help by lending a pair of her own glasses, which helped make the last few weeks of the hospital stay more comfortable.

Throughout the hospital stay, social media and electronic networking presented an option of support for a well-connected woman. She had a strong social network with siblings in 2 states, 3 children, and an extensive group of friends. CaringBridge, a Web site for medical and social updates, was set up by her daughter. It allowed dialogue through feedback and journaling for families. It provided a sounding board for Mike as he shared the emotional ups and downs of the 3-month journey. The CaringBridge reflections are presented later in this article. Barb also used the phone texting function for communication both to her family and members of the health care team, which proved to be a large factor in her anxiety management and regaining control.

DISCHARGE PLANNING

After 3 months in the hospital with a complicated course, the team helped prepare Barb and Mike for discharge to home. Physical therapy focused on stair balance and endurance. Home care services set up home oxygen and remote monitoring. They posed for a tearful picture on the unit, before wheeling out to their vehicle. Both dogs were happily reunited with Barb at home, who continued to recover and gain strength over the ensuing year at home. More than a year later, she has participated in a pulmonary rehabilitation program, weaned from oxygen, normalized pulmonary function testing, and works out at her local health club. She is back working full time and is limited primarily by endurance fatigue and an intermittent dry cough.

The evidence supporting the major challenges with this case study are discussed later: infection, acute lung injury, and progressive mobility.

INFECTIOUS COMPLICATIONS ASSOCIATED WITH NEAR DROWNING

As our case study shows, near drowning can represent a catastrophic event in the life of an otherwise vibrant, healthy patient. Although the major immediate risks of near drowning stem from multiorgan damage and failure caused by prolonged hypoxemia and potential cardiovascular collapse, the infectious complications of near drowning can be severe, and may be associated with more protracted clinical sequelae. Pneumonia is a common and devastating consequence related to the inhalation of contaminated water, particulate matter, and other potentially infectious material during near-drowning events.[1]

EPIDEMIOLOGY

According to surveillance data from the US Centers for Disease Control and Prevention (CDC), drowning was the sixth leading cause of death caused by accidental injury for all age groups in the United States in 2008, with 3548 deaths attributed to unintentional drowning during that year. Drowning was the leading cause of death in children aged 1 to 4 years, and the second leading cause of death in adolescent boys aged 10 to 14 years. In contrast, drowning was the cause of death in only 2.5% of all accidental mortalities among adults aged 40 to 60 years, in 2008.[2] In a year, the CDC estimated that 4174 persons were treated in US hospital emergency departments for nonfatal unintentional drowning injuries, with approximately 53% of these persons requiring hospitalization or transfer for more specialized care.[3]

The incidence of pneumonia associated with submersion injury is unknown because of lack of reliable prospective studies using consistent definitions and population groups. A retrospective study of 125 submersion victims treated at a European ICU cites the incidence of pneumonia in that group as 14.7%,[4] whereas an earlier case series by Oakes and colleagues[5] reported that 16 (40%) of the 40 near-drowning patients in the analysis developed pulmonary infection. Although the true incidence of infectious pneumonia following submersion is difficult to estimate and mortality estimates may be subject to reporting bias, published reports suggest that pneumonia is a complication of near-drowning events.

Although the specific elements predisposing to development of pneumonia following submersion are poorly understood and are likely highly patient specific, several factors are potentially contributory to the likelihood of our patient's progression to pulmonary infection. Both marine and freshwater environments have been shown to possess appreciable contamination by microbial life on sampling for bacteriology.[6,7] Attributes of the body of water itself, such as its temperature and turbulence, contribute to the degree of microbial growth. Warmer standing water tends to be associated with more significant microbial contamination. The volume of fluid aspirated in submersion events ranges from less than 3 to 4 mL/kg seen in most submersion accident survivors to more than 22 mL/kg noted in postmortem studies of drowning.[8] The volume of contaminated water aspirated during a near-drowning event and risk of subsequent pneumonia are likely to correlate, although this has not been studied prospectively. Aspiration of gastric contents and additional particulate material worsens inflammation, permeability, and edema of the airways, increasing the risk of infection by endogenous oropharyngeal microorganisms, as well as by microorganisms from surrounding contaminated water.[1] Any factors that increase the risk of aspiration, the volume of fluid aspirated, or the degree of water contamination during a submersion incident (ie, altered consciousness, precipitating primary event such as a seizure or an arrhythmia, drowning in shallow waters, or stirring up significant particulate material in a struggle during the incident) are all likely associated with higher risks for infectious complications.[1]

DIAGNOSIS AND MANAGEMENT

The diagnosis of pneumonia in the setting of near drowning can be difficult because victims who remain uninfected may manifest signs and symptoms that suggest infection. Fluid aspiration produces radiographic changes that can either mimic or obscure acute infiltrates caused by an infectious process.[1] The development of ARDS can produce a wide variety of clinical symptoms including shortness of breath, rhonchi, and wheezing.[8] Uninfected patients may also develop fever and increased peripheral white blood cell counts, all of which may mistakenly lead to a diagnosis of infectious pneumonia.[9] Microbiologic data can be difficult to interpret because respiratory specimens may reflect high levels of airway contamination during the submersion episode, rather than true infection. The presence of concomitant bacteremia does suggest an invasive infectious process, which may be helpful to the clinician. However, a definitive diagnosis of pneumonia associated with a near-drowning event is difficult to make, forcing the treating team to make a judgment from suggestive clinical evidence alone.

The causative agents of pneumonia following a near-drowning event are varied. Our patient's respiratory cultures were positive for multiple enteric gram negatives such as *Enterobacter*, *Klebsiella*, *Citrobacter* but also multiple organisms that are associated with exposure to contaminated freshwater, namely *Pseudomonas*, *Aeromonas*, *Legionella*, and *Stenotrophomonas* species.[7] As discussed earlier, although the patient did receive a prolonged course of antibiotics, the extent to which each of these microorganisms contributed to the infectious picture in this patient is unclear, because blood cultures were negative and further invasive testing (ie, lung biopsy) was not performed.

However, the patient had multiple subsequent respiratory specimens positive for *Scedosporium prolificans* and *A fumigatus*, concurrent with the development of progressive cavitary infiltrates, and continued dependence on exogenous ventilatory support despite appropriate coverage for bacterial pathogens. Pathogenic molds such as *Aspergillus* and *Scedosporium* (also known as *Pseudoallescheria* species in its sexual form), among others, are prevalent in both the freshwater and seawater environments.[9] Both have been reported to cause pneumonia and other infectious complications in victims of near drowning,[10] sometimes with significant delay in onset of symptoms and clinical manifestations.[9] The patient's clinical course and eventual diagnosis seemed most consistent with fungal pneumonia following a submersion event, for which the patient received a prolonged course of voriconazole, an azole antifungal with activity against a variety of mold species.[11] However, as seen in many cases of near drowning, diagnostic uncertainty can lead to significant antimicrobial exposure for these patients, increasing the risk of untoward consequences such as adverse reactions (ie, dermatitis, allergies) and *C difficile*–associated colitis.

MANAGEMENT OF ACUTE LUNG INJURY ASSOCIATED WITH ARDS

The goal of mechanical ventilation in the setting of ARDS is straightforward: to deliver enough oxygen to the blood to prevent anaerobic metabolism and eliminate enough carbon dioxide to safely control acidosis. Reaching this goal without causing volume or pressure injury to the lung can be challenging. There is controversy about what represents enough oxygen and what equates to safely controlled acidosis. All agree that a normal blood gas is overtreatment in patients with severe lung injury. Life support is the goal as the patient heals from the underlying process.[12]

The severe hypoxemia that accompanies ARDS is the result of air space collapse and filling with edema fluid that provides a path for blood to transit the lung without exposure to air. This shunt cannot be corrected by simply administrating more oxygen to the less severely injured areas of the lung that are still ventilated. Once the hemoglobin in the blood perfusing the ventilated lung is fully saturated, no significant additional oxygen can be added. The only solutions are to minimize the shunt, or perhaps to increase the amount of oxygen in the venous blood.[13]

The ventilator strategies that reduce shunt in acute lung injury are generally referred to as lung recruitment strategies. Positive end expiratory pressure (PEEP) has been used most extensively. The role of PEEP is to prevent end expiratory collapse of injured airways, which not only reduces the size of the shunt but likely reduces ventilator-induced lung injury (VILI) by minimizing recurrent opening and closing of airspace.[14]

There are a variety of ventilator modes intended to recruit airspace while the lung is at near-maximal inflation. Inverse ratio ventilation has a long inspiratory phase matched with a shorter expiratory phase with varying amounts of PEEP. Other strategies are large-volume ventilation and variations of oscillatory ventilation, in which a paralyzed patient is maintained at a high level of CPAP and ventilated with rapid shallow oscillations.[15]

APRV has recently been advocated, although it has not been carefully studied. In this mode of ventilation, a high constant pressure is applied to the lung to inflate it to a projected normal end inspiratory volume. The patient is able to breathe spontaneously over this high pressure, and pressure support can be applied to assist these spontaneous breaths. Every 5 to 10 seconds, there is an intermittent release of the high pressure, which allows a large, rapid ventilator breath, promoting carbon dioxide excretion. The spontaneous breathing that occurs while the lung is inflated likely has beneficial effects on cardiac output and perhaps on the lung itself. There is a reasonable theoretic argument suggesting that the spontaneous efforts may increase the risk of VILI. Large release volumes are avoided, especially given the rapid deflation and inflation times associated with the release breath. The use of alternative ventilation modes such as APRV has not been subjected to randomized clinical trials, and should be done cautiously.[16]

Although most of these interventions improve oxygenation, most have had no proven impact on outcomes and some have been harmful. The balance is that higher pressures and volumes administered to a lung, particularly when it is injured, can harm the lung irreversibly. For instance, large-volume ventilation, greater than 12 mL per kilogram ideal body weight, worsens survival compared with low tidal volume at 4 to 8 mL per kilogram, despite short-term improved oxygenation.[16]

The lung injury that results from ventilation seems to be related to several variables. Large tidal volume/overdistention, high inflating/plateau pressures, and repeated opening and closing of end air space have all been associated with VILI. The rate at which airspace inflates and deflates has also been speculated to be associated with injury.

Although ARDS involves the lung widely, it spares some parts of the lung. In most patients, between 30% and 60% of the lung is normal and can be recruited. However, overdistention of that normal lung can injure it and convert it to nonfunctioning lung. Applying 45 cm of distending pressure to a normal animal lung for 20 minutes (in vitro) causes irreparable injury that is microscopically similar to ARDS. When pressure is briefly applied to heterogeneous lung, the normal lung has a tendency to over inflate and the damaged lung a tendency to remain deflated. This compounds the risk of VILI. The best physiologic support for ideal volume and pressure is based on observations of lung compliance at increasing pressures and volumes. At very low inflation pressures, little or no air enters the atelectatic lung units.[17]

The damage that results from mechanical ventilation probably represents a spectrum from microscopic injury of intracellular junctions resulting in increased pulmonary edema formation, to macroscopic injury of the airways and airspace resulting in intrapulmonary cystic injury, and to rupture of the lung and tension pneumothorax. Our patient probably showed the full spectrum of ventilator-induced injury, but it is often hard to separate the injury caused by the initial illness from that caused by the ventilator.[16]

The best practice for mechanical ventilation in patients with ARDS began with conventional volume-cycled or pressure-cycled ventilator modes with a tidal volume of 4 to 8 mL per kilogram and maximum airway pressures of less than 30 cm H_2O. PEEP should be applied as a primary means of recruiting lung for oxygenation. The arterial blood gas goals are for life support, but not normal values; this is referred to as permissive hypoventilation. Satisfactory levels are typically a pH of 7.20 and a Po_2 of 50 to 55 mm Hg. The hemoglobin saturation goal is 85% to 88%. The Pco_2 is less important in this setting.[17]

Changing from one mode of ventilation to another frequently improves oxygenation with ventilation at least transiently, most likely because of the alteration in flow rates and inspiration and expiration times. Airflow changes slightly from one part of the lung to another. If an earlier mode of ventilation was not working, there may be little else to try. However, there has been little or no convincing evidence that any of the rescue modes of ventilation affect survival. For our patient, the ventilator changes were based on the discussions of the team of physicians and respiratory therapists in collaboration with nurses. Each change produced a different response and adjustment to the plan of care.

Although the various ventilator options are a key part of managing these patients, it is important to recall the role of supportive interventions such as diuresis, antibiotics, moderate-dose steroids, frequent repositioning, and suctioning. These supportive strategies were used for Barb. Inhaled nitric oxide and prostacyclin have been used to increase perfusion of the ventilated lung. Intravenous vasodilators can interfere with physiologic ventilation/perfusion matching reflexes, and are generally avoided.[14] Although there has been controversy about their role, steroids improve oxygenation significantly. It is unclear whether they have a significant effect on survival.[18] The role of neuromuscular blockade is even more controversial, but some modes of ventilator support have frequently required their use. Short-term paralysis almost always results in improvements in oxygenation, but long-term neuromuscular weakness is a frequent complication and survival benefit has not been shown.[14]

PROGRESSIVE MOBILITY

Progressive mobility is advancing each person within their potential to maximize function and reduce risk. Critical care providers have recognized the benefits of less sedation and mobilizing the patient to the extent of hemodynamic stability. Progressive mobility requires the coordinated effort of team members to anticipate and provide for activity needs.[19] Initial activity includes rotation and bed mobility, progressing to mobility out of bed with endotracheal tubes for ventilation. Studies support the benefits of improved oxygenation and early functional recovery with fewer negative outcomes. Increased research has promoted interdisciplinary collaboration and use of devices to improve safe mobility despite tubes and invasive lines.[20,21]

SHARING PERSPECTIVES

The story would not be complete without the perspective from the key persons in this story. Earlier in the article, social media were cited as key communication and healing tools. The following section, written by Mike Smith and family, completes the case presentation.

On the morning of December 3, 2010, the health care/hospital machine opened its gaping jaws and swallowed my wife. For more than 3 months, she was 100% subject to its control every moment of every day. It saved her life. I was an eyewitness to the workings of this awesome machine, and I have been asked to contribute my perspective to this article, as the loved one of a critical care patient.

Two days after Barb was admitted to Rochester General Hospital, our daughter Annie set up a blog on the Web site www.caringbridge.org. This is how the Web site describes its services: "CaringBridge provides free websites that connect people experiencing a significant health challenge to family and friends, making each health journey easier...CaringBridge websites offer a personal and private space to communicate and show support, saving time and emotional energy when health matters most. The websites are easy to create and use. Authors add health updates and photos to share their story while visitors leave messages of love, hope and compassion in the guestbook."

We used this Web site extensively during Barb's hospital stay and beyond. It was a useful way to provide updated information to our family and friends and others, but it also provided me with an outlet that allowed me to verbalize my experience. In all, there were 95 journal posts updating Barb's progress or setbacks, 848 guest entries from family and friends, and 19,484 visits to Barb's Web site. I think the best way for me to describe my experience over the last 14 months is to let our Caring-Bridge posts speak for themselves. What you have just read is what you are probably used to reading in clinical journal articles. What you will now read is how a critical care patient's family processes all of the technical information, deals with the consequences, and copes with them. Every patient and his/her family has this story, varying only with the details.

I will start with my last post, on December 3, 2011, 1 year to the day from Barb's accident.

Saturday, December 3, 2011

One amazing year. One year ago today our lives changed. You were all participants in this amazing experience and the support and love that you showed us in so many ways continues to humble us still. Our last entry was on June 7. I thought that it would be fitting to give you all an update on where we are now, 1 year later. In my last post, I was a wreck because I had just watched Barbara drive down our driveway on the way to a doctor's appointment, by herself. Just last week, Barb drove to Buffalo to pick up Katie at the airport, by herself. Many of you have seen this yourselves, but many have not, so let me tell you that a lot has changed in our lives, and all of the changes have been improvements. Barb works out at our health club 3 to 4 times a week. She is back to work as before, and has regained her control over our checkbook. Thank goodness! There is really not much that she does not do now that she did before, other than tennis and other strenuous activities (not quite there yet). Back in June when I last posted an update, Barb was still on supplemental oxygen 24/7. In July, she gave up the tube during the day; she still used it to sleep because they told us that we do not breathe as deeply when we're asleep. Then, just a couple of months ago, she gave it up completely. The last ornament came off the Christmas tree. There is oxygen paraphernalia in our basement gathering dust, reminding us of darker times and energizing us for the future.

There are small differences; perhaps sometimes they seem less than small, especially to her. Barbara gets very tired at night. That may not seem all that unusual to old farts like us, but it is different. She is still working on her stamina. The day takes a lot out of her. And she has a persistent cough, which I think is the 1 thing that bugs her the most. But they tell us it a sign of healing, so I am happy she coughs, but she is not. Other than that, Barb is Barb. Same wonderful girl but somehow a little bit more wonderful in my eyes. And like I said, the differences are small. The big deal is that Barb is back to being Barb.

As a witness to this healing, I cannot help but be amazed and humbled by my wife's strength and courage. I remember so well the time that she did not have the strength to change the channel on her TV remote. I remember when it was cause for celebration that she was able to get out of bed and walk 2 steps to her chair, with the aid of 2 nurses holding her up! I remember cheering when she told me she had spent 2 straight hours sitting up in her chair. I remember standing there crying with pride as I watched her walk so slowly around the ICU with a walker, pausing to say hello to a nurse or an aide, and then the stern determination on her face that said "I am going to do this lap!"

She did it and was so, so exhausted but defiantly committed. I remember the day she came home from the hospital. It was as much as she could do to climb the stairs to the second floor with my help where I had her walker ready, and she slumped into the walker and I pushed her down the hall to our room because she was so spent. As a mountain climber, I have done many things that left me exhausted, but I realize now that I never even knew the meaning of the word. Now she is walking 5 km or more with the dogs, by herself. She is doing most, if not all, of the things she did before the accident. Barb is back.

I reflect often on this last year. It was so very difficult, indeed the most difficult year I have lived through. I know it was also so for Barb, and also our children. They have had it pretty rough. But on this I will speak only for myself and say that I have never experienced a defining event or line in my life where I can say that before this, I was someone, and after this I was someone else. December 3, 2010, was such a line in my life. So much changed for me. And although it was traumatic and at times terrifying, I look back and think that it was good. I took a long walk today with our dogs and thought long and hard about this, and realized something for the first time. I realized that I see things differently now. It is like viewing something through a fog and all of a sudden you see the same things with a crystal clarity that you have never seen before. It really is almost visual. I see things differently now. So isn't that strange? A terrible, freak accident and many painful months create strength and clarity. What comes out most clearly in this new, focused reality is the strength of our bonds with family and friends, and that is why I am posting this update tonight. I am posting this to thank you. All of you who have been a part of our struggle have been more help to us than you can possibly know. You have changed at least one life, that is mine. And for the better.

Here is how it started, 2 days after the accident:

Sunday, December 5, 2010

When they brought Mom into the emergency room, she was in a coma and intubated. Since then, she has been making slow but steady progress. She has awakened on numerous occasions and seems to recognize family. She has followed instructions (ie, to squeeze my hand) and yesterday even mumbled a few words. Yesterday the doctors attempted to extubate (take out her breathing tube) but she was restless and not getting enough oxygen, although she was breathing on her own. The doctors decided to insert the breathing tubes once again. Today has been a mellow day because Mom is heavily sedated. The doctors are going to give her a few more days to recover and attempt to extubate again.

We will keep you updated if anything changes! We could have never imagined the amount of love and support we have received during this difficult time. Thank you to you all. Annie.

The following are excerpts from journal entries that might give you a sense of how our family responded to and coped with this experience.

Tuesday, December 7, 2010

Today was a day that began with much excitement, but ended with a little disappointment. Barb's pulmonary team was gung ho to extubate her this morning. They expressed the usual provisos, but were excited. They turned down the respirator so that Barb was breathing on her own, and then began the step-down process to bring her to consciousness. She responded well at first, but it became apparent that there was fluid in her lungs, which was problematic. As she continued to do the work (vs the machine), the doctors became worried that, if they took the tubes out and she was unable to cough out the fluid on her own, she would be in trouble. So they took the logical approach and returned her to the status quo. We were disappointed, of course, but realized that Barbara will heal on her own timetable. She had a lot of water in her lungs and that caused injury. The healing process produces fluids. She needs to heal a little more, with help from amazing medical technology and wonderful doctors and staff.

Friday, December 10, 2010

We have had some great news from the nurse this morning that Mom is now following all commands. She is squeezing hands, lifting legs, and moving eyes! She is much more alert than yesterday, which is great.

Friday, December 10, 2010

More great news!! The ventilator is out and Mom is talking to us (although very quietly)! She is able to conduct conversation and everything! She is very tired so she keeps falling asleep. Welcome back Mom!

If I could just say 1 word, it would be Wow! Today has been an amazing day and truly a miracle. When we arrived at the hospital this morning, Mom was awake, very groggy, but awake! The ventilator was out and she was breathing on her own. She can quietly talk to us, and she is even making jokes! She knows who all of us are, and she is so grateful for all of your love and support (we made to sure to tell her).

At the time that Annie posted the update, I (Mike) was in the prep room waiting to be taken into surgery for tendon repair. As I was laying in the hospital bed waiting, a receptionist came up to me and said she had good news. I assumed she was going to tell me that my daughter Katie was on her way back to the hospital. But no, she said that Annie had called and conveyed the amazing news that Barb had awakened. She also said that she was aware of her surroundings, and was talking and following commands. My breath took a hitch and I could not hold back the tears. Even the receptionist started crying. A little later, my anesthesiologist came in to introduce himself and to tell me what to expect. I noticed a large crucifix around his neck, and after he finished, I asked him about the cross and whether he was a religious man. He said indeed he was, so, after I told him about Barb, I asked him if he would say a prayer for her. He was delighted, and proceeded with what was almost a Catholic mass. It was most inspiring and incredibly emotional. As he put me under, I went out with a smile on my face.

We did not know until today whether there had been brain damage caused by the lack of oxygen. this was truly a wonderful day!

Monday, December 13, 2010

We had a setback day today. All of the progress of the last few days is still here; however, there are problems with Barb's lungs that need to be fixed. Without any pulmonary assistance, Barb's lungs are not providing her body with enough oxygen. She has had an assist over the last few days, but apparently during the day today things got worse and they put her on a heavy-duty oxygen mask that provides a real boost of oxygen to her lungs. That mask is a problem for Barb, because it is very uncomfortable and also makes it just about impossible for her to communicate. As all of you know, if Barb is conscious and cannot communicate, that is a big problem for her. The doctors were not sure the mask would work and it might be necessary to reintubate. It seems that the mask is working and we hope that reintubation will not be necessary.

Thursday, December 16, 2010

We are on an episode of House. Everything is so confusing. The results of the tests are not necessarily correlating to her condition, so there must be something else that everyone is missing, and this is what is puzzling the doctors. That being said, the doctors have isolated what is growing in her lungs and have created an antibiotic to attack it. We hoped that this can give Mom some relief, but the doctors still do not know whether it will fix the problem. Mom is currently under sedation and on the breathing tubes. The amount of oxygen that the machine is giving her is slowly being decreased, and she is still able to hold her own. Although this seems disappointing, the doctors have pointed out that it is good news that Mom is not getting worse, in fact she is slowly getting better. It is going to be (and has been) a very long and painful journey, but she will get there.

Tuesday, December 21, 2010

This must be some kind of update record. Do not expect hourly updates going forward, but we just had a very encouraging conversation with Barb's doctor and we thought we should share it with you. Dr Wahl is the chief pulmonologist at Rochester General and one of the most respected in the city. He has been the attending physician since yesterday. He told us that he is very encouraged by Barb's progress and said that he hopes that within 24 to 48 hours, they will be able to take her off the ventilator. He was hopeful last night that they would be able to extubate today, but she had a little episode early this morning when her oxygen level decreased, so they had to increase the machine. She has returned to normal levels, and he is not sure what happened, but thinks it was probably a reaction to one of the many medications she is receiving. Speed bump. Anyway, he likes what he is seeing and uttered the phrase resolution phase, meaning he thinks we're getting close.

This all being said, we have been sorely disappointed in the past and are receiving this news with caution. I would urge you all to do the same.

Thursday, December 23, 2010

Well, we are surely on a roller coaster ride. After the good news from Tuesday, we spoke with Barb's doctor this morning who said, "Well, it hasn't been a great couple of days." Oh man. He said that it has not been a terrible few days, but it is not what we had hoped for. Her lungs are more inflamed than a few days ago, and she has a rash that is spreading. Dr Wahl, Barb's key doctor, was able to explain it to us in a way that made total sense. What he said was that the longer Barbara is in this situation, the more inevitable it is that she will have to deal with issues related not so much to the original problem, but to complications arising from her stay at ICU. Because she is on so much medication, there will be complications arising from the medication itself. His challenge is to figure out a way to cut back on the medications she is on, but at the same time keeping the ones that are helping. It seems to me more art than science. I am not sure whether that worries me or gives me comfort. I think it gives me comfort because I have total confidence in her doctors. They will figure this out. Dr Wahl was honest in that this is a trial-and-error type of project. No one is sure what is helping and what is hurting. That is very frustrating. Once again, it is patience and more patience. The way I look at it is this: it is a miracle that she is alive. So many things could have gone the other way. Just 1 example: cell phone calls from Ellison Park are notoriously inconsistent. I would say it is 50:50 that a call placed from Ellison Park would get through. Hers did. We are truly blessed that she is still here, and I am certain that

Barbara will be back with us soon. Until then, we hope and we pray and we think of her constantly.

Tuesday, December 28, 2010

We had a really nice day today. Barb slept a lot, but was awake enough to have meaningful communications. She is clearly not happy, but who would be? We did not see the doctor today, but Barbara told us (yes, she did) that Dr Wahl was there earlier this morning before we arrived and he performed a bronchoscopy. This information was gleaned through lip reading and word spelling. Pretty cool. Later on, Barbara wanted to know what the results of the bronchoscopy were, but we had not heard anything. This is Barbara getting out in front of her own care. And she can do that without speaking. She is remarkable, as we all know. The previous paragraph shows that the tracheostomy (that is the right word. I have used several, and mangled them all. I plan to enter medical school in the Fall.) has been a godsend for her, and it will only get better. The reason she was so sleepy is because they have been pumping heavy, heavy sedation into her body for 3.5 weeks. That stuff has worked itself into her muscles, skin, and even her bones. Her doctors caution that it will take a while to cleanse out. One other really good thing: once she got those tubes out of her mouth, I was finally able to give her a kiss on the lips. That was really nice for both of us.

Wednesday, December 29, 2010

I have given a lot of thought and consideration to this post. I was sorely tempted to summarize, shorten, and get to the point that Barbara is doing fine. But I realized that you all are in this marathon together with Barb and me and our families, and there is no reason to sugar coat anything. You have gotten the full scoop (almost) to date, so I am going to continue with that. I hope I do not get too stuck in the weeds, but here we go. Around 3:00 AM last night, Barb's right lung suffered an 80% collapse. Staff noticed that her oxygen levels had decreased significantly and she was having trouble breathing. She was immediately taken for a radiograph, which revealed the problem. A chest tube was immediately inserted and it worked. Her lung reinflated rapidly and returned her to the status quo. The reason for the collapse is part of our House episode: apparently she has a small leak in her right lung that, when coupled with the force of the air sent into her lungs by the respirator, was causing a small amount of air to leak into the cavity between the outside of her lung and her rib cage. As this air bubble grew, it began to compete with the lung itself until, eventually, it won and her lung lost. The chest tube, which is an evil-looking contraption with a lot of gurgling fluids doing weird stuff in multiple tubes and blinking lights, did the trick by releasing the pressure from the built-up air bubble, and also releasing some fluid as well, which helped. This procedure allowed her lung to reinflate and regain its normal (hah!) function. (This critical care medicine stuff has really amazed me in its complexity and functionality.)

Thursday, December 30, 2010

First of all, let me say that posting these updates, and then reading your posts later, is very gratifying. I feel like I am speaking to you in a very personal way. I am also trying to convey a little bit of Barb in them. She has not yet had a chance to read them, but will in time. Somehow I think she would want you to know the full story also.

We walked in the room to find a wide-eyed, wide awake, energized very sick person. It was remarkable. She was 100% there. She smiled at us! That is first time I had seen her smile in 3 weeks. My heart was pounding so hard. I could not get this goofy grin off my face.

Barbara was fully engaged and attentive. She wanted to know about my knee.

We had a mini–birthday party with a few gifts. She was touched, excited, and clearly very happy to be celebrating her birthday. I sensed that she understood how special this particular birthday was. Maybe it was just my imagination, but it seemed that she could not stop looking at me. Here is the best. Her respiratory guy Dave (we really like Dave) installed some kind of valve in her wind tube that allowed her to speak! So for maybe 10 to 15 minutes Barbara spoke to us. In her own voice. It was not like that weird metallic sound in the movies. It was her voice. There was not a lot of conversation, but it was wonderful anyway. She liked it too. Oh, and she did this in CPAP, which is doctor-speak for turning the ventilator off. She was on her own, and she did great. There was lots of talk about moving Barb to the Pulmonary Care Unit, which is kind of like graduating from ICU to a less severe environment. Good news.

You cannot believe how much interest and affection Barbara has generated in the ICU in general. So many nurses and aides who have worked with her over the last month have stopped by and checked on her. Some had never seen her conscious. What pure joy and delight we witnessed on their faces to see the real Barbara! Some literally squealed.

Anyway, this post is way too positive. I am excited, and I have allowed this to come through as I write this. This may be a mistake. We know all too well that tomorrow may not be as bright. I am prepared for it, I guess, but I am looking only to the future with optimism and hope. If we are disappointed, and I am sure we will be at times as we continue this journey, then that is just the way it is going to be. We just need to be there for Barbara and support her in any way we can.

Monday, January 3, 2011

Five days in a row! Another good day and another day of pushing limits. When I arrived in Barb's room this morning, her physical therapy aides were moving her from the bed to a chair! It was a recliner, but a chair nonetheless, and she was able to sit up straight with her feet vertical to the floor; this was the first time she had been able to do this since she was admitted. Her face told us that she was clearly a bit scared, especially when she realized that her poor little body could not support its own weight. It was a struggle, but they got her situated and she calmed down. I should mention that she was totally off all respirator assistance, and this was also the first time that this had occurred. The previous CPAP treatment involved a small boost of oxygen at the end of each breath. Now she was totally on her own. I am pleased to report to you all that she sat in that chair and read every single one of your birthday cards. She really enjoyed them all and was clearly moved. By the way, I think there were more than 60 cards! What a great success.

Wednesday, January 5, 2011

Barb had a bit of a setback today, but it was still a very good day. Remember Barb's collapsed lung? Well, it reared up a little bit today. Her chest tube had been removed recently, and they reduced a bunch of other things in the weaning-off process. They noticed a little decrease in oxygenation, so they took a chest radiograph. The leak that was the cause of the original problem apparently is still there; it has improved, but it has not gone. Anyway, by taking out the chest tube, her lung slumped a bit. They put the chest tube back in, and all returned to normal, and then some. It was like last time, everything is working better once they compensated for the leak. Bottom line, her lung is still healing but not yet healed. Her doctor and nurses say it is just a question of time, as usual. Patience…

So the good part was that Barb was up and active pretty much all day. They put the talking valve in her breathing tube and she was able to talk with us for more than an hour. We called Katie, Annie, Anne, Jane, and Susy and they were thrilled to hear Barb's voice come on the line: "Hi Katie!" "Who is this?" "Mom." "Who?" "Mom." "I can't hear what you're saying!" That is when I jumped in. Anyway, it was really good. Barbara was especially excited about being able to communicate freely without the constraints of her dry erase board or lip reading. She told someone "I feel like a new woman."

Thursday, January 6, 2011

Barbara had a mixed day. Her morning was excellent. She inadvertently sat down on her chest tube, which constricted it and caused a minireoccurrence of her lung deflation episode. Maddening, but this kind of thing happens. As soon as they figured it out, she returned to normal but was understandably anxious; she used the right word: scared. That is the reason they gave her the Ativan, which sent her for an afternoon-long snooze, and an afternoon-long setback. Not a big deal, but it irritates me nonetheless. This should not have happened.

Friday, January 7, 2011

Today was another great day for Barbara! Once again, she woke me up by texting me: "When will you be here?" Then I noticed that she had sent me an earlier text at 4:29 AM announcing that "I need lessons…" I later found out she was trying to work the new laptop I had just got for her and was feeling frustrated. Amazing. Lessons? Once again, another good sign for physical therapy.

Sunday, January 9, 2011

A couple of notables. She called me on her phone, and we had an understandable conversation (she wanted to know how to get a DVD out of her laptop). Barb called Katie and talked and talked. She was totally engaged with all of her visitors, and really enjoyed the company. I think was her best day since the accident.

Wednesday, January 12, 2011

I hate, hate, hate to do this. After all, it has been 6 or 7 straight days of progress. But today we had a bit of a backtrack. I have known this was coming; it will come again. But here is what happened today. I got a call from the hospital this morning. Barbara was running a fever (low grade) but worrisome for someone as critical as she is. (By the way, what a wonderful place this Rochester General Hospital is. They are on top of everything! I have so much confidence in the entire team.) Anyway, because of the fever, they did not put the voice box in, so I could not talk to Barb on the phone. Another by the way: it was a pretty big snow storm here in Rochester so I stayed home today (only the second time since the accident I have not seen her). So it was somewhat frustrating to have to communicate by text messages, even more so for Barb. Jumping ahead, her fever cleared around noon. Later, her nurse/practitioner (whom I love) told me that this kind of low-grade fever is very common with patients on long-term tracheostomy. Worry about big things usually resolves to no big deal. What was most disappointing was that her second chest tube did not help. Her lung is still a problem. That needs to change, and they have not figured out the solution yet. We are still getting a lot of "you have to have patience," and "it will take awhile," but I can tell you honestly that it is very, very frustrating to me, but most to Barbara. So we wait, and we remain patient.

We both had a tough day. I mentioned that it has only been twice since December 3 that I have not been with her. We also have not been able to talk on the phone, which I have kind of gotten used to. I know, I am spoiled; texting is a really inferior way to communicate. Also, it is tough when we have seen so much progress, and now another speed bump. Patience, patience…

Thursday, January 13, 2011

So, around 4:15 PM, her wonderful nurse Margaret came in and we asked about the radiograph results. Margaret told us that the pictures showed a "smidge" of improvement, which, by reading body language, clearly disappointed her doctors (Margaret explained that a smidge is a very technical medical term that we probably would not understand). But Margaret told us this: "I told the doctors that I have been in this business for 30 years and I don't care what the x-rays show. I know from watching her for the last 4 hours that she is better. She is stronger, her voice is stronger, she looks better. Something good is happening." So let us hope that dear Margaret is right. I know exactly what she is talking about though. Barbara looked really good this afternoon.

One other thing before I go. Unlike before, Barbara knows that you all are out there and are pulling for her, praying for her, wanting her to get better. She makes sure that she reads the CaringBridge updates and guestbook logs every day, and she appreciates it more than you can possibly know. I watch her read a post, and she just shakes her head slowly like she cannot believe this, and a little tear forms. You are helping; she hears you and she really loves what she hears. I really think it helps in her recovery. I know you want to hear from her, and you will. She is just not quite ready for that. I jumped the gun, I have to admit.

Saturday, January 15, 2011

We left around 2:00 PM and went to watch Annie's boyfriend Eric in a track meet at the Rochester Institute of Technology. All the while, I was texting Barb and asking how she was doing but not getting any response. I was worried. Then later I went out for a beer with my friend Jason and still had not heard from Barbara, until eventually my phone buzzed and she was sending me text messages: "Are you out with Jason?" "Are you OK?" "Please text me to let me know you are OK." These rapid-fire texts came all in the space of about 3 minutes. I had been trying to raise Barbara for 4 hours! Anyway, it ends up that she had been asleep for the last 4 hours, and now, guess what, she feels really good. So, back to emotions. I was worried, and upset, and nervous almost all day. Now I am flying high. I know this is a long-term process that requires patience and more patience, but I still cannot avoid feeling overly worried, and then, as now, probably overly euphoric. I have got to learn to settle down. I am not sure it is possible, but I am going to work on it.

Monday, January 17, 2011

This morning started well enough for Barbara. She slept pretty well, had physical therapy in the morning, which went very well, and then her visitors started to arrive. All in all, she was great; active, with it, and feeling pretty good.

Later, around 3:00 AM after Barb and Annie had left, Margaret came in and said she had been thinking over the weekend and wanted to give something a try. (I have mentioned Margaret before on these pages. I do not know how to nominate someone for sainthood, but I would if I could.) She explained patiently to Barbara what she wanted to do, and then she did it. She removed the oxygen line from Barb's tracheostomy and capped it, essentially shutting it down. She then attached an oxygen line into her nose to give her a little more O_2 than normal air.

This made a really big difference. She was visibly more comfortable, and she said so. She is essentially breathing on her own, and, most exciting, Margaret speculated with fingers crossed that maybe, just maybe, this week they could remove the tubes. Barbara of course told her to shut up and not get her hopes up, but the reality is that today was a major movement from one plateau to the next, or, as Margaret put it, she passed over a major hump today with flying colors. We will see what tomorrow brings, which of course may be a reversal, but right now things look really bright. Speaking of which, Barb just called me (at 8:00 at night!) and we discussed (mostly) her concerns about me. Regardless, it was obvious she felt really good, which most assuredly is attributable to Margaret's experiment today.

Another potentially positive development: if all continues well, as it has all day, there is a good chance that they will be able to remove 1 of her chest tubes tomorrow. I think progress is shown by the removal of those Christmas tree ornaments from her body. Soon, she will be able to eat real food, drink real orange juice. She is already breathing on her own and her tracheostomy tubes have been rendered inactive. Folks, I think Barbara is getting there.

Tuesday, January 18, 2011

This will just be short and sweet. They left Barb's tracheostomy tube capped all night last night and all day today. Graduation. She passed her swallow test and is now able to eat. Graduation. They removed 1 of her chest tubes (the first one they installed) because it had done its job. Graduation. By the way, that particular tube was causing Barb serious discomfort (pain) that they did not realize it was the problem until it was gone. Hurray!

Barb called me at least 3 times today just to chat or because she had a question for me. Seemed pretty normal, which feels odd. What a great treat to see her cell phone number come up. I had missed that.

Barbara is now on the formal Rochester General Hospital meal plan! She had a tuna fish sandwich and apple sauce for lunch, then meatloaf tonight. I do not think she ate too much. The flavors (such as they were) kind of overwhelmed her. Just image this: you have not tasted anything for 6 weeks, and now you taste tuna fish? A bit too much, I am thinking. Anyway, what an improvement, and she will get used to it and start to receive nutrition that she has not been able to get until now, which will expedite her healing.

Wednesday, January 19, 2011

Barb and I had a very gratifying conversation with Margaret today. She reminded us that for more than 6 weeks, Barb has been in critical shape. Everything that her medical team did, every treatment, every recommendation, was focused on her survival. The idea of returning to normalcy was not part of the conversation. Margaret smiled when she said that now it is different. Now the medical, dietary, and rehabilitative judgments and recommendations that they are making are focused on getting Barbara back to where she was before the accident. That is a fundamental shift in approach, and an acknowledgment that she is getting better, and better, and better. Barb convinced Margaret that it would be OK for me to bring her a turkey sandwich from home. She was pleased about that. She reported that the meat at dinner last night was more akin to shoe leather than beef and it made it very difficult to get her nourishment. A turkey sandwich sounded pretty good to her.

Thursday, January 20, 2011

I thought this update is worthy of a special post this morning. Barb's tracheostomy is out! Gone! No more tubes!

Very, very exciting!

Tuesday, February 1, 2011

Barbara woke up this morning with a new attitude. Phrased bluntly, it was: "I'm getting the hell out of here. Let's get to it!" She was up and out of bed, sitting in her chair, by 8:00 AM. She had a shower and a shampoo, and did her physical therapy like a champ. She felt better, stronger, actually pretty good. Margaret said she was intrigued by this new focus, and very excited. She knows better than most that recovery is very much a mental and emotional battle. Barbara seems to have turned somewhat of a corner in that regard. She had been frustrated, disappointed, and tired. At least today, she was positive, determined, and committed. I am excited. I asked her whether she was going to wake up tomorrow with the same attitude, and she immediately said, "Absolutely!"

Friday, February 4, 2011

Real short update tonight. Barb had a good day. Lots of energy and she felt pretty good. She had a really long nap this afternoon, which bugged her, but she probably needed it. As Tony noted, she has gained almost 2 kg in the last 2 weeks, which is really good. She walked, on the arm of her nurse (but without the aid of a walker, I might add) to her bathroom for a shower this morning, which is great progress. Barb has mentioned several times recently that she feels like she is getting stronger. I can see it in her face, in her voice, and in her general demeanor. She ate more tonight (hospital food no less; no McDonalds) than I have seen her eat since she was able to eat. That is another very good sign.

Yesterday, when Stephanie and Nancy were visiting with Barb and her new best friend Margaret, the subject of cruises came up. You see, Stephanie just had her 50th birthday and her sisters treated her to a surprise cruise out of Miami for a few days. Nice! Anyway, the gals got chatting and the subject of cruises came up, and why one would want to do that or not. Margaret said that she would not want to go on a cruise because it cost a lot of money, and what if the weather was bad, or she got sea sick; what a waste of money! Barbara responded that the reason she would not spend the money on a cruise was that she worried that she might get legionnaires' disease. What a jokester.

Now Barb chimes in for the first time. This took her at least 2 hours to write:

Saturday, February 5, 2011

Dear family and friends and friends of family and friends, it is me, Barb! I have been listening (my family would read to me) and more recently reading your entries. I cannot tell you how much your words of encouragement and inspiration have helped me deal with this overwhelming situation. I have heard my everyday friends, from friends I have known since nursery school. Thank you so much for taking the time to speak to me...I hear every word. Also, thank you to everyone that brought food to our house. I heard I missed some good food. Also, thank you so much for all of your cards, they make my day when I receive them. And then there is my family. My kids are there for me every day by phone or daily visits from Jack; that is one way to have quality time with your 20 year old, although I would not recommend this approach.

My dear, dear Mike. He has been my rock and everyday cheerleader. I cannot imagine going through this without him. I am feeling stronger every day. My biggest obstacle is the healing of my lung. With your continued support, it will help me face the upcoming challenges. I did not plan on this being so long, but I have so many things and people to be thankful for. Thanks from the bottom of my heart!

Love, Barbara.

Monday, February 7, 2011

Today was a pretty exciting day. I went to see Barbara a little early and was privileged to see a day in the life of my dearest wife. I had not seen her do physical therapy for a few weeks. She seemed a little reluctant to jump into it when her physical therapy coach arrived, but she was game. Expecting not much, she got up out of the chair, walked 10 steps forward with the walker, turned around, and walked back. Sat back down and rested a little. Then she did it again. Most impressive! But it was even better: she did not really get winded, and her oxygenation level stayed very high. Nice. She seemed very pleased.

Thursday, February 10, 2011

The Barbara/Chance and Sammy (our 2 golden retrievers) reunion went off without a hitch. Jack and I drove the boys to the hospital, and we met just outside an entrance. Annie and Eric were there also. The dogs were so excited but also very distracted by all the confusion. Both hopped up into Barb's lap. She enjoyed the visit very much, and so did they. Trouble is, they are clearly confused. They acted somewhat morose the rest of the day. "Why doesn't she come home?" They do not understand. On a different level, neither do I. It was a busy day for Barb and, by late afternoon, she was pooped.

Friday, February 11, 2011

Today was a big day folks! The chest tube is gone! One last ornament off the tree. Finally untethered after 10 weeks to the day. She feels good, her O_2 numbers are great, she is doing very, very well. Barb's physical therapy was strong this morning. The only negative thing that happened today is that she was unable to take a shower because she could not get the area where the chest tube was inserted wet. Oh well. Barb, Jack, and I had a pizza party in her room tonight (I even smuggled in a beer!) Although it was still a hospital room and a bit clinical, it was almost festive. What a great development today!

Tuesday, February 22, 2011

On her walks through the Pulmonary Care Unit, the physical therapist or nurse walks behind Barb pushing her chair so that, if she gets tired or winded, she can just sit down and rest. On Saturday, as Barb was starting her walk, her nurse was getting the chair arranged and she looked up and Barb was almost out of the room. She said "Barb, can you please slow down?" It was pretty funny. Then as she strolls through the unit, she receives enthusiastic greetings from the entire staff. "Hey Barb! You go girl." She responds to everyone with a friendly greeting and a smile. Sometimes she even waves. Barbara has made a lot of friends (and fans) at Rochester General Hospital.

There have also been a few downs. On Sunday night, Barb awoke around midnight with a very rapid heartbeat, around 200 bpm. She was given a drug that immediately slowed it down, but they took blood and otherwise worked on her for quite a while. As a result, she did not sleep much the rest of the night and was pretty exhausted all day yesterday. The cardiologist said that she might be experiencing subventricular tachycardia (SVT). This is the second time she has had this kind of episode since she has been in the hospital. It is not particularly dangerous, but it is not really a good thing. It also can cause (drumroll please) dizziness and fainting. They are not sure that this is the cause, and more tests (electrocardiogram, and so forth) are going to be performed. If it is SVT, that could explain a lot. It is also treatable; indeed, several world-class athletes (like the guy who came in third in the 1998 Tour de France) have had it with no ill effects. As a result of this development, moving Barb to a rehab facility has been put on hold pending test results, and so forth.

Saturday, February 26, 2011

We have been having several conversations with Margaret about a very exciting subject: going home! Barb's strength and stamina are improving to such an extent that we can actually envision the prospect. Although there are no firm discharge plans at this point, we are starting to think about what would be involved and what we would have to do to make it work. We are of course very excited, but it is also a bit scary. The plan is to wait and see how the electrophysiology study goes, and then make some decisions. It seems as though we are about to enter the next phase of this amazing ordeal. Three months! It is hard to believe.

Sunday, March 6, 2011

I have been waiting for more than 3 months to post this update, and I do so with great joy and gratitude. Barbara is scheduled for discharge on Tuesday; she will be coming home. There is a whiteboard in her unit that I see every day when I visit and that is labeled Discharge. It lists the names of the patients who are scheduled to be discharged in the next 2 days. Until last week, it was difficult to conceive of the day when B. Smith would be on that list. Tomorrow, I will see her name on the board.

I want to say here that I have never been prouder of anyone in my life. Barbara responded to this massive assault resulting from terrible luck with strength I have never seen. Although suffering from pain, frustration, disappointment, and agony I could not have imagined had I not witnessed it, she never felt sorry for herself. She hardly even complained. She has treated her caregivers with gratitude and respect, appreciating all that she was being given, which of course was her life. I have never been in her presence when she did not say thank you to a nurse, aid, doctor, or technician who did something for her. She has been an amazing example of strength, grace, and humility.

Tuesday, March 8, 2011

Here is the shortest and best update yet: Barbara is home!!

There was a lot more that was posted to Caring Bridge after Barb's return home, but suffice it to say that it was a story of progress and improvement. The operative word from the beginning was patience, and that is the overall take-away from this. Our story was one of patience, waiting for Barb to heal, waiting for things to get better, and they have. Two weeks ago, Barb's pulmonary doctor advised us that her lungs were functioning at 81% capacity. That is on the low end of normal, but in the normal range. In late June, 2011, her lungs were at 40%. To be where she is now was inconceivable just months ago.

Things are not back to normal. Barb continues to have a persistent cough, which could be permanent. She is not back to normal aerobic activity yet and probably will not be for months. However, she still attacks her rehab and physical training with a vengeance, determined that she will return to where she was before the accident. She is positive, optimistic, and determined.

Barb is an inspiration to us all, especially to me. Her strength in the face of this calamity was inspiring, and continues to be so. I believe that we all have it in ourselves to be this strong, but she was able to succeed only because of what the machine was able to do. The term machine may connote a negative, but I do not intend to convey that. The machine that I am talking about was a lifesaver. The important thing to understand is that this machine comprised individuals, many, many individuals, who made the difference and who saved Barbara's life. I will never, ever forget you. Thank you from the bottom of my heart.

SUMMARY

Although this was a prolonged hospital stay, the positive outcome of survival to resume function buoyed teams across the continuum of care. This case offered many learning opportunities for our team. Progressive mobility helped limit the reconditioning and supported her recovery. Strategies for chest tube management to allow safe mobility included extra length, labeling, and ample space to move. Coordination of care among providers helps with selection of the best ventilation modes. Keratitis may have been avoided if the initial check in the emergency department/ICU included assessment of the presence of contact lens. Social media supported communication and allowed discussion of feelings, loss, and change. Our hospital team partnered with a loving family to share our story.

REFERENCES

1. Gregorakos L, Markou N, Psalida V, et al. Near-drowning: clinical course of lung injury in adults. Lung 2009;187:93–7.
2. Centers for Disease Control National Center for Health Statistics (NCHS). Injury prevention & control: data & statistics. Available at: http://www.cdc.gov/injury/wisqars/index.html. Accessed December 20, 2011.
3. Gilchrist J, Gotsch K. Nonfatal and fatal drownings in recreational water settings - United States, 2001–2002. MMWR. Available at: http://www.cdc.gov/mmwr/preview/mmwrhtml/mm5520a7.htm. Accessed March 29, 2012.
4. Van Berkel M, Bierens JJ, de Rooy TP, et al. Pulmonary oedema, pneumonia, and mortality in submersion victims: a retrospective study in 125 patients. Intensive Care Med 1996;22:101–17.
5. Oakes DD, Sherck JP, Maloney JR, et al. Prognosis and management of victims of near drowning. J Trauma 1982;8:123–5.
6. Auerbach PS, Yajko DM, Nassos PS, et al. Bacteriology of the marine environment: implications for clinical therapy. Ann Emerg Med 1987;16:643–9.
7. Auerbach PS, Yajko DM, Nassos PS, et al. Bacteriology of the freshwater environment: implications for clinical therapy. Ann Emerg Med 1987;16:1016–22.
8. Olshaker JS. Submersion. Emerg Med Clin North Am 2004;22:357–67.
9. Garzoni C, Garbino J. Long-term risk of atypical fungal infection after near-drowning episodes. Pediatrics 2007;119:417–8.
10. Katragkou A, Dotis J, Kotsiou M, et al. Scedosporium apiospermum infection after near-drowning. Mycoses 2007;50:412–21.
11. Cecil JA, Wenzel RP. Voriconazole: a broad-spectrum triazole for the treatment of invasive fungal infections. Expert Rev Hematol 2009;2:237–54.
12. Gattinoni L, Protti A, Caironi P, et al. Ventilator-induced lung injury: the anatomical and physiological framework [review]. Crit Care Med 2010;38(Suppl 10):S539–48.
13. Esan A, Hess DR, Raoof S, et al. Severe hypoxemic respiratory failure: part 1-ventilatory strategies. Chest 2010;137:1203–16.
14. Fan E, Wilcox ME, Brower RG, et al. Recruitment maneuvers for acute lung injury: a systematic review. Am J Respir Crit Care Med 2008;178:1156–63.

15. Tang BM, Craig JC, Eslick GD, et al. Use of corticosteroids in acute lung injury and acute respiratory distress syndrome: a systematic review and meta-analysis. Crit Care Med 2009;37:1594–603.
16. Myers TR, MacIntyre NR. Respiratory controversies in the critical care setting: does airway pressure release ventilation offer important new advantages in mechanical ventilator support? Respir Care 2007;52:452–8.
17. The Acute Respiratory Distress Syndrome Network. Ventilation with lower tidal volumes as compared with traditional tidal volumes for acute lung injury and the acute respiratory distress syndrome. N Engl J Med 2000;342:1301–8.
18. Dreyfuss D, Saumon G. Ventilator-induced lung injury: lessons from experimental studies. Am J Respir Crit Care Med 1998;157:294–323.
19. Needham D. Mobilizing patients in the intensive care unit improving neuromuscular weakness and physical function. JAMA 2008;300:1685–90.
20. Fitzpatrick M, Vollman K, Swadner-Culpepper L, et al. Progressive mobility in the critically ill. Crit Care Nurse 2010;30:S1–16.
21. Hopkins RO, Spuhler VJ, Thomsen GE. Transforming ICU culture to facilitate early mobility. Crit Care Clin 2007;23:81–96.

Index

Note: Page numbers of article titles are in **boldface** type

Crit Care Nurs Clin N Am 24 (2012) 625–631
http://dx.doi.org/10.1016/S0899-5885(12)00091-3
0899-5885/12/$ – see front matter © 2012 Elsevier Inc. All rights reserved.

ccnursing.theclinics.com

Moving?

Make sure your subscription moves with you!

To notify us of your new address, find your **Clinics Account Number** (located on your mailing label above your name), and contact customer service at:

Email: journalscustomerservice-usa@elsevier.com

800-654-2452 (subscribers in the U.S. & Canada)
314-447-8871 (subscribers outside of the U.S. & Canada)

Fax number: 314-447-8029

Elsevier Health Sciences Division
Subscription Customer Service
3251 Riverport Lane
Maryland Heights, MO 63043

*To ensure uninterrupted delivery of your subscription, please notify us at least 4 weeks in advance of move.

United States Postal Service

Statement of Ownership, Management, and Circulation
(All Periodicals Publications Except Requester Publications)

1. Publication Title	2. Publication Number	3. Filing Date
Critical Care Nursing Clinics of North America	0 0 6 - 2 7 3	9/14/12

4. Issue Frequency	5. Number of Issues Published Annually	6. Annual Subscription Price
Mar., Jun, Sep., Dec	4	$144.00

7. Complete Mailing Address of Known Office of Publication (Not printer) (Street, city, county, state, and ZIP+4®)

Elsevier Inc.
360 Park Avenue South,
New York, NY 10010-1710

Contact Person: Stephen R. Bushing
Telephone (Include area code): 215-239-3688

8. Complete Mailing Address of Headquarters or General Business Office of Publisher (Not printer)

Elsevier Inc., 360 Park Avenue South, New York, NY 10010-1710

9. Full Names and Complete Mailing Addresses of Publisher, Editor, and Managing Editor (Do not leave blank)

Publisher (Name and complete mailing address)

Kim Murphy, Elsevier, Inc., 1600 John F. Kennedy Blvd. Suite 1800, Philadelphia, PA 19103-2899

Editor (Name and complete mailing address)

Katie Hartner, Elsevier, Inc., 1600 John F. Kennedy Blvd. Suite 1800, Philadelphia, PA 19103-2899

Managing Editor (Name and complete mailing address)

Adrianne Brigido, Elsevier, Inc., 1600 John F. Kennedy Blvd. Suite 1800, Philadelphia, PA 19103-2899

10. Owner (Do not leave blank. If the publication is owned by a corporation, give the name and address of the corporation immediately followed by the names and addresses of all stockholders owning or holding 1 percent or more of the total amount of stock. If not owned by a corporation, give the names and addresses of the individual owners. If owned by a partnership or other unincorporated firm, give its name and address as well as those of each individual owner. If the publication is published by a nonprofit organization, give its name and address.)

Full Name	Complete Mailing Address
Wholly owned subsidiary of	1600 John F. Kennedy Blvd., Ste. 1800
Reed/Elsevier, US holdings	Philadelphia, PA 19103-2899

11. Known Bondholders, Mortgagees, and Other Security Holders Owning or Holding 1 Percent or More of Total Amount of Bonds, Mortgages, or Other Securities. If none, check box. ☐ None

Full Name	Complete Mailing Address
N/A	

12. Tax Status (For completion by nonprofit organizations authorized to mail at nonprofit rates) (Check one)
The purpose, function, and nonprofit status of this organization and the exempt status for federal income tax purposes:
☐ Has Not Changed During Preceding 12 Months
☐ Has Changed During Preceding 12 Months (Publisher must submit explanation of change with this statement)

PS Form 3526, September 2007 (Page 1 of 3 (Instructions Page 3)) PSN 7530-01-000-9931 PRIVACY NOTICE: See our Privacy policy in www.usps.com

---

13. Publication Title			14. Issue Date for Circulation Data Below
Critical Care Nursing Clinics of North America			September 2012

15. Extent and Nature of Circulation			Average No. Copies Each Issue During Preceding 12 Months	No. Copies of Single Issue Published Nearest to Filing Date
a. Total Number of Copies (Net press run)			628	558
b. Paid Circulation (By Mail and Outside the Mail)	(1)	Mailed Outside-County Paid Subscriptions Stated on PS Form 3541 (Include paid distribution above nominal rate, advertiser's proof copies, and exchange copies)	396	346
	(2)	Mailed In-County Paid Subscriptions Stated on PS Form 3541 (Include paid distribution above nominal rate, advertiser's proof copies, and exchange copies)		
	(3)	Paid Distribution Outside the Mails Including Sales Through Dealers and Carriers, Street Vendors, Counter Sales, and Other Paid Distribution Outside USPS®	76	77
	(4)	Paid Distribution by Other Classes Mailed Through the USPS (e.g. First-Class Mail®)		
c. Total Paid Distribution (Sum of 15b (1), (2), (3), and (4))			472	423
d. Free or Nominal Rate Distribution (By Mail and Outside the Mail)	(1)	Free or Nominal Rate Outside-County Copies Included on PS Form 3541	52	45
	(2)	Free or Nominal Rate In-County Copies Included on PS Form 3541		
	(3)	Free or Nominal Rate Copies Mailed at Other Classes Through the USPS (e.g. First-Class Mail)		
	(4)	Free or Nominal Rate Distribution Outside the Mail (Carriers or other means)		
e. Total Free or Nominal Rate Distribution (Sum of 15d (1), (2), (3) and (4))			52	45
f. Total Distribution (Sum of 15c and 15e)			524	468
g. Copies not Distributed (See instructions to publishers #4 (page #3))			104	90
h. Total (Sum of 15f and g)			628	558
i. Percent Paid (15c divided by 15f times 100)			90.08%	90.38%

16. Publication of Statement of Ownership

If the publication is a general publication, publication of this statement is required. Will be printed in the December 2012 issue of this publication. Publication not required.

17. Signature and Title of Editor, Publisher, Business Manager, or Owner

Stephen R. Bushing – Inventory Distribution Coordinator   Date: September 14, 2012

I certify that all information furnished on this form is true and complete. I understand that anyone who furnishes false or misleading information on this form or who omits material or information requested on the form may be subject to criminal sanctions (including fines and imprisonment) and/or civil sanctions (including civil penalties).

PS Form 3526, September 2007 (Page 2 of 3)

Printed and bound by CPI Group (UK) Ltd, Croydon, CR0 4YY

03/10/2024

01040460-0008